The safe, healthy way to lose body fat and keep it off —
PERMANENTLY.

How To Lose Body Fat

With this easy-to-read book, you'll find:
- Simple ways to measure excess body fat
- Tailor-made diets, menus, and recipes
- Special exercises for a double-reducing effect

"Before you try one more diet . . . you need this book."

> *Fred L. Allman, Jr., M.D.*
> Former Chairman,
> American Medical Association's
> Physical Fitness Committee

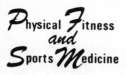

Physical Fitness and Sports Medicine

Below is a listing of the currently available (or soon to be available) books in this new series:

- *Strength-Training Principles* by Ellington Darden, Ph.D.
- *Olympic Athletes Ask Questions About Exercise and Nutrition* by Ellington Darden, Ph.D.
- *How to Lose Body Fat* by Ellington Darden, Ph.D.
- *Soccer Fitness* by David Ponsonby, M.Ed., and Ellington Darden, Ph.D.
- *How Your Muscles Work: Featuring Nautilus Training Equipment* by Ellington Darden, Ph.D.
- *Care and Conditioning of the Pitching Arm* (For Little League Baseball) by Fred L. Allman, Jr., M.D.
- *The Week-End Athlete's Guide to Sports Medicine: Lower Body* by James D. Key, M.D.
- *Nutrition For Athletes* by Ellington Darden, Ph.D.
- *Conditioning For Football* by Ellington Darden, Ph.D.
- *The Week-End Athlete's Guide to Sports Medicine: Upper Body* by James D. Key, M.D.

Write to Anna Publishing for a complete description of titles, publication dates, and prices.

Anna Publishing, Inc.
Post Office Box 218
Ocoee, Florida 32761

How To Lose Body Fat

Ellington Darden, Ph.D.

Director of Research
Nautilus Sports/Medical Industries
Executive Program Director
Athletic Center of Atlanta, Georgia

Anna Publishing, Inc.

Contents

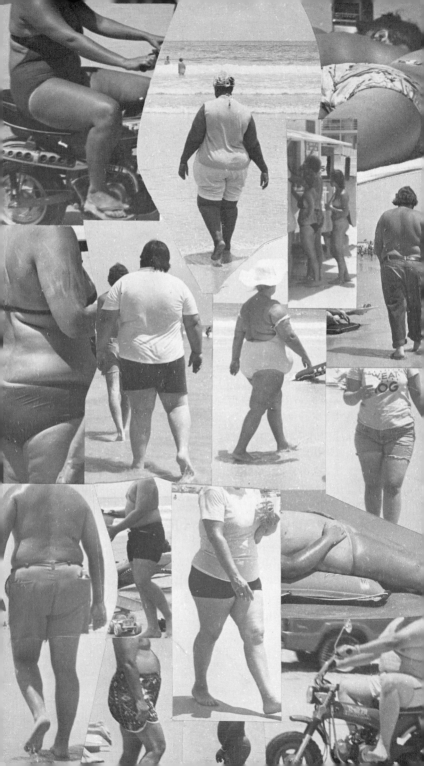

Preface

The words **weight** and **fat** are frequently used in discussing the human body. Yet these terms are often misunderstood.

For example, let's examine the concepts of body weight, body fat, overweight, and over-fat.

Body weight is simply what your entire body weighs . . . the amount of skin, bone, muscle, fat, etc. you have from head to toe . . . which can be recorded in pounds or kilograms. This is usually measured on pressure- or balance-type scales.

Body fat is composed of three types of fat: subcutaneous (directly under the skin), depot (inherited storage areas), and essential (around vital organs). Each type will be discussed in more detail in Chapter 2; however, let me briefly say that your total body fat can not be measured as accurately as your body weight.

Overweight is a term that in recent years has been determined by referring to the popular height-weight charts. Most of these charts have descended from averages of men and women who had bought life insurance policies between 1885 and 1908. Even though they've been updated, many questions still arise as to their accuracy.

For example, what about the variance of your weight depending on the time of day, the season, your clothing, and your state of digestion? Or what about your body build? Do you have a large, medium or small frame? If you have wide hips, how do you know if the extra width is from bone or fat? And what about your ethnic background? As you should realize by now, the concept of overweight really leads to more misunderstanding than understanding.

Over-fat is an idea that can be particularly meaningful to most people. Over-fat can be defined as a bodily condition marked by excessive deposition and storage of fat. The key word is fat! It's not unusual to see people who are within the desirable ranges of the height-weight charts and are still over-fat. Or they can be overweight and not over-fat, or underweight and actually over-fat. It all depends on the amount of muscle and the amount of fat that you have on your body.

On the one hand, the major function of muscle is to move our bodies. The more muscle we have, the stronger we are, and the more efficiently we move. The average American man or woman, therefore, would benefit from having more muscle.

On the other hand, the major function of fat is the long-term storage of energy . . . which is both good and bad. Good if we are stranded on a desert island with little food. Bad if we live in America where food is plentiful, where slimness is idolized, where sports participation is in vogue, and where there are little or no opportunities to get stranded on a desert island! Most people in this country would be more efficient and healthier if they significantly reduced their body fat.

It's estimated that at least two billion pounds of excess fat are being carried on the bodies of the American people. Each year these individuals spend more than 10 billion dollars searching for an answer to this problem. Most of the so-called "answers," unfortunately, are ineffective or even dangerous.

How to Lose Body Fat was written specifically to provide sensible, scientifically-based solutions to over-fat problems . . . solutions that produce results, dramatic results. While this book is certainly useful to coaches, trainers, and athletes, it's primary usefulness will be to middle-aged Americans . . . middle-aged Americans who want to lose body fat, and middle-aged Americans who want to remain lean and healthy.

Are you an over-fat American? Do something about it today!

A microscopic view of human body fat tissue.

Chapter 1
Before: Over-Fat and
Out-of-Shape

Sammy Johns, Martha Hunter, and John Kalas have never met, yet they have a great deal in common. I have a suspicion that when you read about them you'll find that you have a lot in common with them, too.

Sammy Johns

"For as long as I can remember," said Sammy, "I've loved to eat. During the last several years,

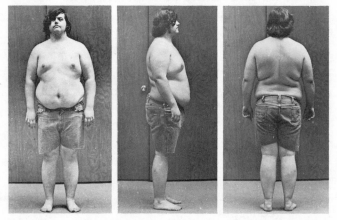

When these photos were taken of Sammy Johns, he was 22 years of age and weighed 299 pounds, at a height of 6 feet.

I've become addicted to a nightly ritual of watching TV, eating cheese and crackers, and drinking beer. It's not unusual at all for me to consume two pounds of cheese, two boxes of saltine crackers, and a case of beer (24 bottles) ... all in a single night of TV watching." And on top of this, he could sincerely look you in the eyes and say: "Doesn't everyone eat cheese and crackers and drink beer when they watch TV?"

When Sammy wasn't watching TV or eating, he was assembling exercise machines at the Nautilus plant in Lake Helen, Florida. That's where I met him four years ago. After several months of my verbal abuse mixed with encouragement, Sammy agreed to let me put him on a low-calorie diet and progressive exercise program.

Sammy Johns had lived in a small town all his life. Since he did very little reading, he had no preconceived ideas about losing fat (fad diets) or proper exercise. As a result, he did **precisely** what we told him to do -- no more, no less! He was the perfect pupil.

Problems
- Majority of food consumed at night
- Little or no nutritional knowledge
- No idea of proper exercise

Solutions
- Working knowledge of basic nutritional concepts
- Memorize four basic food groups

- Understand guidelines for selecting three, low-calorie meals a day
- Supervised, high-intensity exercise three times a week

Martha Hunter

In 1974 and 1975, I worked very closely with Dr. Fred L. Allman in his Sports Medicine Clinic in Atlanta, Georgia. It was during this period of time that I met Martha Hunter.

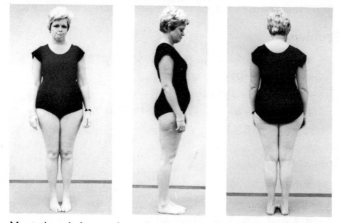

Married and the mother of two teenagers, 42-year-old Martha Hunter was 5' 4" in height and weighed 148 pounds.

"I was just plain tired of looking at my flabby body," said Martha with a bit of skepticism in her eyes. "And since I've tried every diet and exercise program on the market at least twice, I might as well give your method a try."

Martha is typical of many women in that they know they are fat, and they are motivated to do something about it. But each time they successfully lose 10 pounds, they promptly revert to their old habits. Soon they're back where they started.

One of Martha's biggest problems was her week-end habits. She could stick to a diet perfectly during the week. The social gatherings on Fridays and Saturdays, however, were her downfalls.

In other words, Martha kept trying to modify her dietary habits, when what she really needed was a drastic change, rather than a modification. In order to make this change, Martha Hunter needed frequent supervision and encouragement.

Problems

- On again, off again dietary practices
- Willing to try anything
- Lack of confidence
- Needed to be vigorously pushed in diet and exercise

Solutions

- Specific, day-by-day dietary guidelines to follow
- Patience and discipline
- Weekly exercise goals

John Kalas

In January of 1976, John Kalas (a prominent pathologist in DeLand, Florida) phoned us at the Nautilus plant. Dr. Kalas was interested in the effects of high-intensity exercise on reducing blood cholesterol levels.

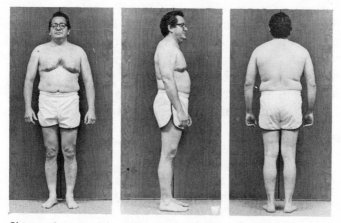

Shown above is John Kalas, M.D., Head of the Department of Pathology at West Volusia County Hospital. At 45 years of age, Dr. Kalas was 5' 8" in height and weighed 220 pounds.

Several weeks after I started Dr. Kalas on an exercise program, I realized he was also concerned about his own over-fat condition.

Listen as John explains: "At a height of 5' 8" and a weight of 220 pounds, I knew my health was in a state of dangerous decline. At 45 years of age, I was a prime candidate for a heart attack. No one knew the cardiovascular risk factors as well as I did. Yet, I just couldn't find the time to exercise. My daily routine consisted primarily of sitting activities: sitting in my car, sitting behind a microscope, sitting at my desk, and sitting at the dinner table. What I needed was a sensible and quick exercise and dietary program -- something that produced results -- something that I could practice and become positively addicted to!"

Dr. Kalas was a highly motivated person. He had been a successful athlete in his high-school days. And although he was an above average tennis player, he couldn't help but think that his valuable time could be better spent in a more demanding and challenging activity. As a result, he was in a constant state of turmoil and tension . . . a human time bomb ready to explode.

Problems

- Erratic eating patterns
- Too busy, not enough time to exercise
- Tense, highly motivated personality

Solutions

- Three small, low-calorie meals a day
- Brief, high-intensity exercise three times a week
- Learn to relax

Basically, all three of these people had similar problems: (1) overeating (their weekly energy intakes exceeded their weekly energy outputs), and (2) underactivity or improper exercise.

Sammy's dietary and exercise program was carefully monitored for six months. Martha's training was carried forth over a three-month period of time. John's program took 12 months. Later in this book you'll be given details on how to organize your own three-month, six-month, or twelve-month dietary and exercise program . . . a program that's guaranteed to produce significant losses in body fat. (For those of you who just can't wait to read the **how-to's**, the "after" photos of Sammy, Martha, and John are shown in Chapter 9.)

Before you get overconfident, however, let me warn you: losing body fat is not easy and it is not quick! On the contrary, losing body fat is hard, very hard . . . and it takes time . . . and patience . . . and discipline . . . and motivation . . . and know-how!

For every individual who successfully loses body fat, and keeps it off . . . there are hundreds of others that try and fail. Why? Simply because they can't profit from their own mistakes . . . or the mistakes of others.

Don't let yourself fall into these categories. Make up your mind today, that three months from now, and six months from now, and twelve months from now . . . there's going to be a new, leaner, healthier, and better looking YOU!

Chapter 2
What is Body Fat?
How is it Measured?

Most of your body fat is composed of subcutaneous fat and depot fat. Subcutaneous fat consists of layers of fat found directly under the skin all over the body. It makes up the major percentage of fat in most individuals. Depot fat, on the other hand, while often more conspicuous than subcutaneous fat, makes up less of total fat content. It is usually deposited in the abdominal region in men and around the hips and thighs in women.

In addition to the two categories of fat mentioned above, a third type is called essential fat. This is the fat that is essential to the normal maintenance of the body. It makes up the covering of nerves, the membranes of cells, and cushions and protects many vital organs of the body.

If we take a male of average frame with a correct body weight relative to height (according to the tables that many insurance companies use), that person would have approximately 16 percent body fat. An average female subject fitting the same requirements, however, would have approximately 26 percent body fat. This is due to the larger percentage of subcutaneous fat that most females have developed, primarily as a result of genetics and hormones. It's important to keep this in mind when trying to determine your body fat status. For example, the onset of obesity is usually considered to be 20 percent body fat in males, but 30 percent in females.

Please note the frequent use of the word "approximately" in the above statements. Whenever height and weight alone are used to make assumptions about percent body fat, we are treading on thin ice. It's quite possible for an individual to be overweight by the height-weight charts, and not be over-fat. Or a person could be underweight by the charts and actually be over-fat.

How can you determine your percentage of body fat? There are numerous scientific techniques that could provide you with specific answers. Each of these techniques, however,

Skinfold calipers can be used to measure the thickness of your subcutaneous fat. The calipers, however, are rather difficult to obtain as they must be ordered from medical laboratories at a cost of over $100. This photo shows a 12 millimeter measurement being taken from the mid-triceps area of the upper arm.

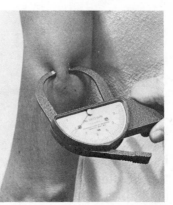

from skinfold calipers . . . to underwater weighings . . . to total body potassium, has certain shortcomings.

From a practical point of view, general fatness can be determined by simply looking into a full-length mirror. An honest appraisal of the nude body can be a reliable guide for locating excessive body fat . . . especially the fat that is stored directly under the skin. While viewing yourself in the mirror, you can roughly determine your fat storage spots by pinching various parts of your body.

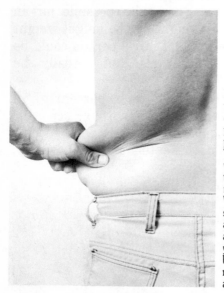

Fat directly under the skin can be estimated by pinching various parts of your body. The sides of the waist are one of the first places that men store fat. Women tend to store fat first around their thighs and hips. One of your goals should be to bring that fat roll down to half an inch or less.

For example, pick up a pinch of skin from the back of your arm, midway between the elbow and the shoulder (mid-triceps area). You should have a double layer of skin and fat, excluding the

To estimate your fat, pinch and measure a double layer of skin from the following seven areas: front thigh, back thigh, hips (upper buttocks), waist (front and side), back (over shoulder blade), and upper arm (mid triceps). More than three quarters of an inch thickness on a male's body or one inch thickness on a female's body indicates excessive fat in that area.

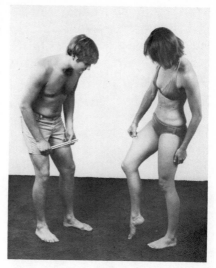

underlying muscle, between your thumb and forefinger. When you take your fingers away, have a ruler handy so you can measure the distance between your fingers (to the nearest eighth of an inch). Most parts of your body can be pinched and measured in this fashion. Generally speaking, more than three quarters of an inch thickness on a male's body or one inch thickness on a female's body, indicates excessive body fat. You can expect these rough measurements to naturally vary, with greater figures indicating your inherited patterns of fat distribution.

One last suggestion for those of you who are really interested in losing body fat. Put on a snug bathing suit and have a good friend take some full-length photos. That's right . . . photos of you from the front, side, and back . . . similar to the ones I've used in Chapter 1. Now when you have

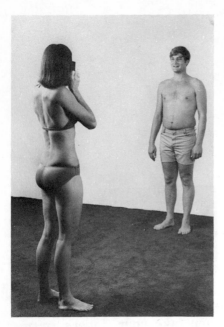

Full-length photographs are a great motivational tool for the over-fat individual. For best results, be sure to stand in front of an uncluttered background in a relaxed manner.

the film developed, request that two prints be made of each negative.

When the prints are returned, take one set of photos, write your weight and the date on the back, and put it away for safe keeping . . . you're going to need it for comparison purposes later. Then, select the worst one of the remaining group (the photo in which you look the fattest) and carry it around with you, in your billfold or pocketbook, every day . . . wherever you go. Look at it often, especially before meals and before retiring. Let the photograph remind you of your present state of fatness. And let the photograph motivate you to do something about it . . . NOW . . . and every day hereafter!

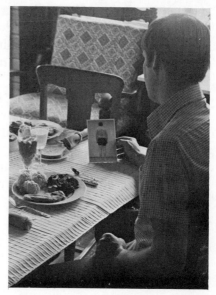

As a reminder of your over-fat condition, look at your "before" photographs often . . . especially prior to each meal.

With all our over-fat and out-of-shape subjects, we try to update our full-length photographs at least once every six weeks. It would be well worth your time and effort to do likewise. It's very motivating to see your fat-loss results in pictures as well as on the scales. You should have quite a fascinating visual record after four or five months.

The primary portion of your fat-loss program will consist of well-balanced, low-calorie meals. Chapters 6 and 7 contain the necessary guidelines for you to plan meals that will get results.

Although there are many fine points involved in the effective application of the simple rules of caloric restriction and nutritional balance, they're everything that sound medical and nutritional science has to offer for the management of obesity at this time. No wonder so many people seek a way out of this difficult-to-accept reality and turn to some **fad, crash,** or **magic** diet formula instead.

To help convince you of the logic behind well-balanced, low-calorie meals, it is necessary to understand some of the **illogical reasoning** behind the various unbalanced, fad diets . . . and over-the-counter reducing gimmicks. The next two chapters should help clear the air.

Chapter 3
Fad Diets

All diets, balanced or unbalanced, "fad" or "crash," will produce weight loss (but not necessarily fat loss) if the total calories they provide in 24 hours amount to less than your total caloric requirement for weight maintenance. Certainly weight loss will appear to be somewhat

At your local book store, you can find all kinds of diet and nutrition books. Can you recognize the books that are sensible and scientifically-based from those that advocate fads and fallacies?

faster on some diets than on others. But no diet will result in the loss of fat if it ignores the principle of conservation of energy and the first law of thermodynamics by not providing for significant calorie restriction.

Probably the most misleading type of fad diet is that which permits unlimited consumption of certain high-protein foods. Examples are the "Calories-Don't-Count Diet," which adds safflower oil to unlimited proteins and fats with very little carbohydrate; the "All-The-Meat-You-Want Diet;" and "The Doctor's Quick Weight Loss Diet" allowing unlimited amounts of certain meats, fish, eggs, and cheeses and requiring ingestion of at least 8 glasses of water daily.

The life span of each of these diets is brief because it takes at most a few days or weeks for the people misled into following them to discover that they cannot continue. The reason for the failure of these diets is simple enough: **they run counter to the basic principles of balance, minimal change, and the teaching of good dietary habits for permanent control.**

After a short period of time on one of these diets, you're only able to force down a limited amount of calories. As a result, you frequently do lose weight -- simply because as you become bored with eating the same foods you actually reduce your calories.

Another type of fad diet may require some caloric restriction but demands either a sharp reduction of carbohydrate intake or no carbohydrate at all. An example is "The Drinking Man's Diet," which substitutes alcohol for carbohydrates. Alcohol contains little or no nutrients but calories.

Other diets of this type have been cloaked in a mantle of respectability by such names as, "Mayo Clinic Diet" -- a name that has been applied over the years to more than a dozen diets, none of which had the frailest connection with this renowned institution. Similarly, the so called "Air Force Diet" has been emphatically disowned by the Air Force.

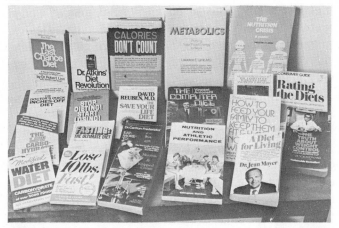

What are some good books to add to your food and nutrition library? The nine books on the right of the middle are highly recommended and are listed in the bibliography. The books to the left are *not* recommended.

And let's not forget the most famous of the low-carbohydrate diets: "Dr. Atkins' Diet." In this diet, carbohydrate intake is reduced to 60 grams or much less, while fat and protein are usually unlimited. The "scientific" explanation being offered for the alleged effectiveness of

27

low-carbohydrate diets is that in the fat person carbohydrate is rapidly converted to fat tissue, rather than being used for energy, whereas calories from fat and protein are burned up in the metabolic processes and aren't stored as body fat. **This is simply not true.**

What does appear to be true to some extent is that excess calories from whatever source are less readily utilized and more readily stored in the fat person. **The initially greater weight loss resulting from a low-carbohydrate diet providing the same number of calories as a balanced, mixed diet is actually due to an additional loss of body water, not fat.** Ignorance of this scientifically proven fact has probably led to more confusion in the dietary treatment of obesity than any other single factor.

To understand this, a strong differentiation must be made between fat loss and scale-weight loss. The scale measures total weight only -- and cannot distinguish fat loss from water loss or loss of vital lean tissue. A diet that contains carbohydrates, but is well below your caloric requirement in total caloric content, will produce a reduction in scale weight that will parallel fat loss for only a few weeks. Then, although your body fat continues to decrease, retention of water will set in and mask or counter balance the fat loss. If the diet contains little or no carbohydrate, this apparently disturbing phenomenon doesn't occur.

Yet carbohydrate must be furnished in the diet, despite this disadvantage, for a number of compelling reasons. First of all, if lifetime calorie control is to be acceptable, the diet must have some palatability and appeal. Much of the variety and taste in foods are furnished by carbohydrates. In addition, carbohydrate is an essential nutrient although not quite as indispensable as certain of the amino acid constituents of protein. Your body has a specific need for carbohydrate as a source of energy for the brain and for other specialized functions. The Food and Nutrition Board of the National Research Council has suggested that the normal adult requires approximately 500 carbohydrate calories daily.

Another category of fad diets is those that are low or inadequate in protein. An example is the greatest crash "diet" of all time, "total fasting." Here you are given only non-caloric liquids and of course, no protein. Other examples of the low-protein diet are the "Rockefeller Diet," the "Grapefruit Diet," the "Skimmed Milk and Banana Diet," and the "Doctor's Quick Inches-Off Diet."

Adequate protein intake is a basic requirement for health. A reducing diet, just like a normal diet, must contain sufficient protein to maintain the body structure. If this isn't furnished in the reducing diet, the vital need has to be filled by the breakdown of your body's lean, non-fat, protein tissue. Most of this will come from muscle and some of it from organ tissue. Naturally this is **physiologically undesirable.**

Chapter 4
Over-the-Counter
Reducing Gimmicks

Despite the efforts of the pharmaceutical industry, no satisfactory fat reduction drug has been developed. In other words, you will not lose fat simply by consuming a certain capsule, tablet, or pill.

This does not, however, stop your local drug store from carrying these products. These so-called reducing pills offer "a wonderful kind of plan to get rid of 5, 10, 25, or more pounds of unsightly fat. Not by suffering thru starvation dieting hunger . . . not by sticking to boring reducing diets . . . not by extra tiring exercises." These products (according to their manufacturers) are "for people who love to eat."

The package of the reducing aids may mention a plan as well as the pills. It may say "Bioslim T with diet plan" . . . "Prolamine with diet plan" . . . "Ayds reducing plan candy" . . . or even call the package "Appedrine diet reducing plan," but no more is said about the plan on the outside of the package. On the inside, however, there are sometimes booklets -- some as long as 42 pages of print so small it is almost unreadable -- advising that the only way to lose weight is to eat less. Eating less means being on a diet and, in fact, the plans advise a highly restricted caloric diet.

People who purchase these "reducing aids" are paying very high prices and at best buying a diet, the sort available in most women's magazines. The profit margins on appetite control products, according to the November 1975 **Chain Store/Drug Edition,** is up to 45 percent. The sale of these products expands by better than 20 percent per year. Sales this year are expected to hit at least 90 million dollars. They are among the fastest growing group of items in drug stores today.

What is contained in these expensive and ineffective products? The Food and Drug Administration's Over-the-counter Panel of Miscellaneous Internal Drug Products has divided them into three categories:

(1) those containing a combination of benzocaine, methylcellulose, and sucrose (such as Slim Mint, Unitrol Chewing Gum, and Slim Line Candy)

(2) those with a combination of phenyl-propanolamine (PPA) and caffeine (such as Bioslim T, Prolamine, Caldrin, Appedrine, and X-11 tablets)

(3) those with alginic acid, sodium carboxy-methylcellulose, and sodium bicarbonate (such as Pretts and Ex-Calorie Wafers).

Other products contain varying combinations of the above ingredients. Ayds is in a category by itself because it is simply a candy with vitamins.

All the products claim to control appetite and hence induce weight loss.

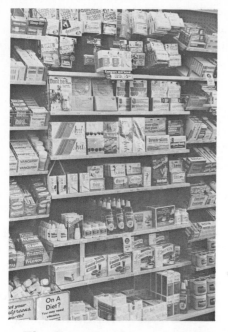

The nation's chain drug stores are expected to sell over $90 million worth of appetite control products this year. Very few of the over-the-counter products help you to lose fat in the long run.

The diuretics (drugs that increase the secretion and flow of urine) sold over-the-counter are very weak and produce a slight loss of water. They produce no loss of fat at all. They have been poorly studied in terms of side effects, but it is safe to say that if they produced dramatic weight loss, they would do it by dehydration, which can be dangerous if the person has heart, liver, or kidney disease. They should not be used for the treatment of obesity.

Propanolamine is an amphetamine-like drug with all the advantages and disadvantages of amphetamines, except that the over-the-counter

32

products have very small quantities of the drug . . . not enough to produce therapeutic or toxic effects. Amphetamines are not recommended because they produce only transient appetite suppression and they are addictive. The same can be said for propanolamine. In well-controlled studies of more than two years' duration, propanolamine has not been shown to cause fat loss.

The bulk producers are supposed to give you a feeling of fullness and diminish the appetite. No long-term studies have shown their efficiency. A person could just as likely produce this result by eating a lot of carrots.

Benzocaine is supposed to anaesthetize the taste buds so that food doesn't taste good. Again, there's no good scientific evidence to support the claim of sustained fat loss.

The candy-type appetite weight suppressants again have not been demonstrated to be effective in long-term, well-controlled trials.

Dr. James Ramey, Clinical Professor of Medicine at George Washington Medical School, states flatly that all the over-the-counter weight loss/appetite control claims are nonsense and lies. He says, "The laws of thermodynamics hold for humans; matter is neither created or destroyed. The only way to lose fat is to eat fewer calories than your body burns. None of the over-the-counter products aid in dieting in the long run. Until they can be shown to be effective, they should be withdrawn from the market."

In summary, the most these over-the-counter products can do is serve as a psychological crutch

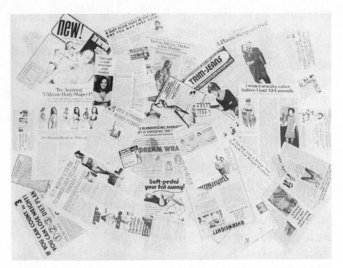

The photo above shows a montage of diet and exercise advertising that was recently taken from popular magazines. Contrary to what these ads would have you believe, there is no quick and easy way to lose body fat.

to help a dieter eat less. **Buying reducing pills will help you lose money, but not fat.**

Before getting to the requirements for nutritionally balanced, low-calorie diets, let's briefly touch on some factors that influence the storing and losing of body fat.

Chapter 5
Factors that Influence Body Fat

Basal Metabolic Rate

This refers to the rate that your body uses energy to maintain itself during a state of complete rest. Your body's regulator for the basal metabolic rate is thyroxin, a hormone secreted by the thyroid gland. If there's a deficiency in the amount produced, a lower metabolic rate will result, thus reducing the total caloric requirement. Conversely, an overproduction of thyroxin will increase metabolic activity and caloric expenditure. Malfunctioning of the thyroid and other glands, however, appears to play only a minor role in the problem of obesity. In one study of 275 obese individuals, less than three percent had a glandular disorder that could be blamed for their problems.

Efficiency of the Digestive System

There's a definite variability in the digestive systems of individuals and their ability to break down the energy component of food. An individual with an efficient system is able to supply the body with more calories from the same amount of food than an individual with an inefficient system. This creates the need for a greater expenditure of energy through activity or a lower intake for an equal amount of work. Digestive system efficiency is difficult to determine without extensive medical tests.

Appetite Regulating Mechanism

Generally speaking, appetite is thought to be controlled by a part of the brain called the hypothalamus. The hypothalamus is sensitive to the amount of sugar in the blood; low sugar levels produce stimulation of appetite. Some authorities, however, think the appetite of an obese person is more attuned to the **sight, smell**, and **taste** of food than that of the non-obese person.

Fat Tissue Cell Size

The fat cells in the obese person are often increased in number as well as size, **particularly if the obesity began in childhood or is of extreme degree.** Thus a greater number of fat cells means an increased cell mass, even when individual cells are normal in content. If an obese individual mobilized fat from these normal-sized but more numerous fat cells, he would still have a relatively large mass of fat cells containing relatively little fat. This would constitute a barrier to weight reduction because, while fat cells can be created, they cannot be destroyed.

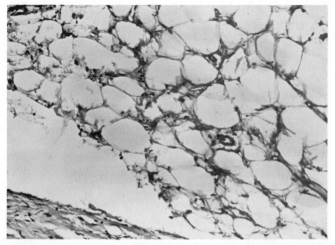

This photo shows fat cells intermingled with connective tissue. You can increase the size and number of fat cells, but you can only decrease the size of fat cells, never the number. In other words, it's much easier to prevent obesity than treat it!

Heredity and Environment

Studies have shown that three out of four obese individuals come from families with a history of obesity. Whether this tendency toward obesity is caused by hereditary factors or by acquired family eating habits hasn't yet been clearly determined. Although heredity is a possible factor, the more likely cause seems to be the development of the overeating habit from family and culturally instilled attitudes. In some families, preparing and serving a continuing array of attractive, usually high-calorie meals is considered an expression of love rather than a means of providing needed nourishment for the body. Another culturally developed attitude that can lead to overeating is one that insists "the plate must be cleaned." Overeating habits developed from such attitudes and patterns instilled from early childhood are difficult to break.

Emotional Overeating

Emotional and personality factors are often interwoven with obesity, and they are remarkable for their complexity and diversity. When lonely, frustrated, bored, or unhappy, some people turn to food for psychological release. In many respects, it's similar to alcohol, smoking, or drug addiction. Also, this tendency is often developed from early family practices of using food as a "reward" for good behavior or as a means of consolation during times of illness or other difficult times.

Water Retention

In some persons, particularly women, a distressing factor in efforts to control weight is a tendency toward excessive water retention. The condition is called **edema** or bloating, and has nothing to do with calorie intake or expenditure. Edema in women quite often begins just before the menstrual period and continues throughout the period. During such times or for those with a more persistent problem, the elimination of certain foods such as salt, pickles, salted butter, salted or cured fish and meats, and crackers can be helpful. For those with special water retention problems, a variety of diuretics may be prescribed by a physician.

Chapter 6
Nutritional Requirements
for a Balanced Diet

It should be evident that fat loss by dieting can be accomplished by caloric reduction. The best way to restrict your food is by actually counting calories. In doing this, however, two precautions must be taken: (1) an adequate food calorie chart or predetermined total calorie meal plan should be used, and (2) the diet must adequately meet the nutritional requirements of the body.

The three major classes of nutrients that your body requires are carbohydrates, proteins, and fats. Other nutrients include vitamins and minerals.

The foods necessary to supply all the nutrients for the repair, growth, and energy needs of the body are classed into four major groups: meat, milk, fruits and vegetables, and breads and cereal.

Meat Group

Included in this group are meat, fish, cheese, beans, dry peas, eggs, nuts, and poultry. These foods are all high in protein and ample amounts of fat. Daily intake should include two or more servings, preferably with each meal supplying some protein from these sources.

Milk Group

Adults do not outgrow their need for dairy products (at least two servings a day are needed). This group includes whole and skimmed milk, buttermilk, yogurt, cottage cheese, ice cream, and cheese. Protein, fat, and calcium are all found in dairy products.

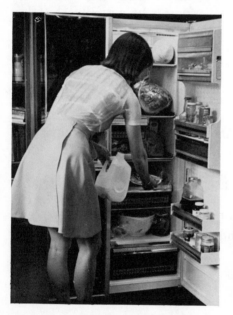

Milk or dairy products and fresh fruits and vegetables should always be an important part in any well-balanced, low-calorie meal.

Fruit and Vegetable Group

Servings from this group should amount to three or four a day, with both green and yellow fruits and vegetables included. Fruits and vegetables are excellent sources of carbo-hydrates, vitamins, and minerals.

Bread and Cereal Group

This group includes enriched or whole-grain breads and cereals. Three or four servings should be included each day. Though the primary contribution of this group is carbohydrate energy, it also contains protein, vitamins, and minerals.

Other Foods

Most foods have serious functions to perform . . . the jobs of building, maintenance, and repair. But what of other foods, like candy, soft drinks, butter, margarine, salad dressings, and snacks? Should they be written off or sacrificed? As long as the basic nutritional needs are attended to, everyone should have access to this group . . . at least a limited access.

All foods in this group are primarily sources of energy; some like butter or margarine, contribute vitamin A. By themselves, they cannot nourish and sustain you, but they do add flavor and variety to meals, satisfy appetites, and add to the joy of living.

There is danger, however, when these "extras" get out of hand (when they are eaten excessively, or when they crowd out important protective foods). When large amounts of fat must be lost,

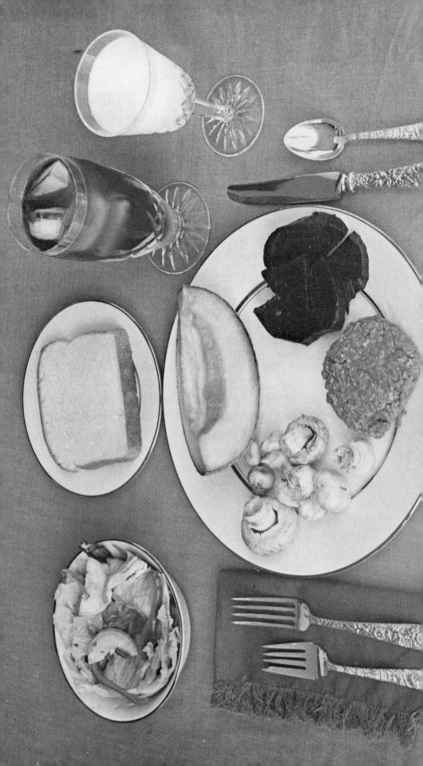

DIETARY GUIDELINES FOR LOSING FAT
(Sample Diets)

FOOD	FOR 1,200 CALORIES DAILY	FOR 1,500 CALORIES DAILY	NOTES
Meat Group	3 small servings (or a total of 7 ounces cooked weight)	3 small servings (or a total of 7 ounces cooked weight)	Choose lean, well-trimmed meats: beef, veal, lamb, pork. Poultry and fish should have skin removed. One egg can be substituted for 1 serving of meat.
Milk Group	2 cups fortified skim milk	2 cups whole milk	Two cups milk means two 8-ounce measuring cups.
Fruits and Vegetables Group	4 servings	4 servings	One fruit serving = 1 medium fruit, 2 small fruits, 1/2 banana, 1/4 cantaloupe, 10-12 grapes or cherries, 1 cup fresh berries or 1/2 cup fresh, canned or frozen unsweetened fruit or fruit juice. Include one citrus fruit or other good source of vitamin C daily.

One vegetable serving = 1/2 cup cooked or 1 cup raw leafy vegetable. Include one dark green or deep-yellow vegetable or other good source of vitamin A at least every other day. |

NOTE: Because of space limitations, calorie tables are not included in this book. There are many inexpensive, paperback books that provide this information. One such book is prepared by **Consumer Guide Magazine** and is listed in the bibliography.

FOOD	FOR 1,200 CALORIES DAILY	FOR 1,500 CALORIES DAILY	NOTES
Bread and Cereal Group	4 servings	5 servings	One serving = 1 slice bread; 1 small dinner roll; 1/2 cup cooked cereal, noodles, macaroni, spaghetti, rice, cornmeal; 1 ounce (about 1 cup) ready-to-eat unsweetened iron-fortified cereal.
Other Foods	1 serving	3 servings	One serving = 1 teaspoon butter, margarine, or oil; 6 nuts; 2 teaspoons salad dressing; or 35 calories or less of another food.

this group of foods is the first and best place to make your cuts.

The preceding chart, based on selections from the Four Basic Food Groups, should be useful to all dieters. With this chart, you'll find guidelines for 1,200- and 1,500-calorie diets.

Some dieters don't want general guidelines. They want specifics: which foods, how much, and how often. If you fall into this category, then Chapter 7 is tailor-made for your needs and wants. In it you'll find a 30-day, 1,000-calorie-a-day diet that's well balanced from head to toe. All you have to do is read, understand, and obey!

Chapter 7
Low-Calorie
Menus and Recipes

Warning! Anyone who has ever become seriously obese will always be a prime candidate -- even after successful fat reduction -- for rapid reversion to his previous over-fat condition. The sensible dietary guidelines that I've described in Chapter 6 and the low-calorie menus and recipes that follow, should teach you what to eat and how to eat for the rest of your life.

The key to losing body fat is the strict adherence to a diet that is restricted in calories but balanced in terms of nutrient content.

"Calories" and "balance" . . . these are the key words. A fat-reducing diet that is centered around these concepts is the only suitable one for the treatment of obesity. Why is this true? Because all that is needed to make it a proper balanced diet for maintenance -- as opposed to reduction -- of weight is an increase in the size of food portions. In other words, after you successfully lose the unwanted body fat, you are also prepared with the necessary guidelines to control these problems in the future.

On the following pages, you'll find 30 days of menus . . . menus totalling approximately 1,000 calories each day. (Recipes for the numbered foods are listed at the end of the chapter.) For best results, you'll want to weigh or measure most of the food portions . . . at first, anyway. And don't skip any meals. Everything's been tested and tried for total nutrition.

Low-Calorie Menus

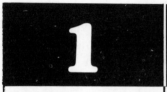 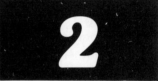

BREAKFAST, 210 calories: 1 orange or ½ cup orange juice; 1 egg (large) cooked to own preference (soft boiled, poached, or fried in no-calorie vegetable cooking spray); 1 slice low-calorie bread or toast; 1 teaspoon low-calorie margarine or 1 tablespoon low-calorie jelly; no-calorie beverage (coffee, tea, water, soda).

LUNCH, 400 calories: Summer Salad[1]; 1 slice low-calorie bread; 4 oz. turkey; ½ cup skim or low-fat milk.

DINNER, 400 calories: ¼ cup cottage cheese; ½ cup asparagus; ¼ cup cooked carrots; 1 slice whole wheat bread; ½ cantaloupe or honeydew melon; 4 oz. leg of lamb, lean; no-calorie beverage.

  TOTAL CALORIES: 1,010

BREAKFAST, 270 calories: Grilled Swiss cheese sandwich; 1 oz. Swiss cheese; 1 tablespoon low-calorie margarine spread on 1 side of 2 slices low-calorie bread, grill using no-calorie vegetable spray; 1 cup tomato or V-8 juice; no-calorie beverage.

LUNCH, 360 calories: 4 oz. lean ground hamburger; 1 slice low-calorie bread; 1 peach or plum; ½ cup boiled broccoli with 1 table- spoon lemon juice; no-calorie beverage.

DINNER, 370 calories: ½ cup skim or low fat milk; 1 slice low-calorie bread; 10 raw or steamed oysters (medium size), coctail sauce, 2 tablespoons; baked apple; ½ cup cooked peas; no-calorie beverage.

  TOTAL CALORIES: 1,000

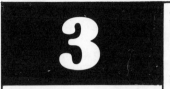

3

BREAKFAST, 210 calories:
1 oz. cold cereal or ⅓ cup
(uncooked) oatmeal; ½ cup
skim milk or low fat milk;
½ grapefruit or ½ cup grapefruit juice; no-calorie
beverage.

LUNCH, 395 calories:
4 oz. roast beef on 2 slices
low-calorie bread with 1 teaspoon mustard; ½ cup
asparagus; ½ cup straw-
berries; 1 oz. farmer or pot
cheese; no-calorie beverage.

DINNER, 375 calories:
4 oz. roasted turkey, meat
only; ½ cup broccoli, with 1
tablespoon lemon juice;
1 slice rye bread; ½ cup
cooked beets; ½ honeydew
or cantaloupe melon;
no-calorie beverage.

TOTAL CALORIES: 980

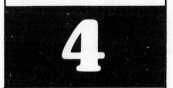

4

BREAKFAST, 205 calories:
½ cup fresh diced pineapple;
1 slice honey ham loaf; 1 slice
low-calorie bread or toast;
1 teaspoon low-calorie
margarine or 1 tablespoon
low-calorie jelly; ¼ cup

cottage cheese; no-calorie
beverage.

LUNCH, 385 calories:
3½ oz. tuna fish (oil packed,
drained); ½ cauliflower,
boiled or raw; 1 slice low-
calorie bread; 1 banana;
½ cup skim or low fat milk.

DINNER, 410 calories:
4 oz. roast beef, lean; 1 baked
potato, without skin; 1 tablespoon sour cream; 1 slice
low-calorie bread; ½ cup
strawberries; no-calorie
beverage.

TOTAL CALORIES: 1,000

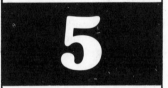

5

BREAKFAST, 255 calories:
French Toast[2]; 1 teaspoon
low-calorie margarine or
1 tablespoon low-calorie jelly;
½ cup apple juice; no-calorie
beverage.

LUNCH, 315 calories:
Spinach Salad[3]; 2 tablespoons Italian low-calorie
salad dressing; 1 slice
pumpernickel bread; 1 teaspoon low-calorie margarine;
2 slices bacon cooked crisp;
5 prunes (dried); no-calorie
beverage.

DINNER, 425 calories:
4 oz. veal loin chop for Veal
Parmesan[4]; ⅓ cup tomato
sauce; ½ oz. Mozzarella
cheese; ½ cup cooked

cabbage; ¼ cup fresh sliced pineapple; ½ cup skim or low-fat milk.
TOTAL CALORIES: 995

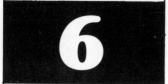

BREAKFAST, 250 calories: Dominique Egg[5]; 1 orange or ½ cup orange juice; 1 small sliced tomato; no-calorie beverage.

LUNCH, 370 calories: Honeydew-Turkey Salad[6]; ½ cup cauliflower with paprika; 1 slice whole wheat bread; ½ cup skim or low-fat milk; no-calorie beverage.

DINNER, 380 calories: ½ cucumber, sliced; ¼ cup cottage cheese; 4 oz. flounder filet, with 1 tablespoon lemon juice; 1 slice rye bread; 1 ear of corn (medium size); 1 teaspoon low-calorie margarine; 1 apple; no-calorie beverage.
TOTAL CALORIES: 1,000

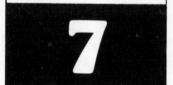

BREAKFAST, 235 calories: 1 cup tomato or V-8 juice; ½ cup flavored yogurt; 1 slice of low-calorie bread or toast; 1 teaspoon low-calorie

margarine or 1 tablespoon low-calorie jelly; no-calorie beverage.

LUNCH, 355 calories: Beef Patty Parmesan[7]; Mushroom Parsley Salad[8]; no-calorie beverage.

DINNER, 405 calories: ½ cup skim or low-fat milk; 4 oz. roasted chicken, meat only; 1 cup spinach cooked with 2 tablespoons vinegar; 1 slice whole wheat bread; ¼ cup unsweetened apple sauce; no-calorie beverage.
TOTAL CALORIES: 995

BREAKFAST, 265 calories: 1 oz. cold cereal or ⅓ un-cooked oatmeal; ½ cup skim or low fat milk; 1 banana; no-calorie beverage.

LUNCH, 370 calories: Cucumber-Tuna Salad[9]; 2 carrots in sticks; 1 slice pumpernickel bread; 1 cup strawberries; ½ cup skim or low fat milk; no-calorie beverage.

DINNER, 365 calories: ½ can beef consomme'; 1 frankfurter; ½ cup cooked onions; 1 slice low-calorie bread; ½ cup mashed acorn squash; ½ cup grapes; no-calorie beverage.
TOTAL CALORIES: 1,000

9

BREAKFAST, 215 calories:
1 cup strawberries; 1 egg (large) cooked to own preference; 1 slice low-calorie bread or toast; 1 teaspoon low-calorie margarine or 1 tablespoon low-calorie jelly; no-calorie beverage.

LUNCH, 370 calories:
¾ cup cottage cheese; ½ cup green beans (boiled or raw); 1 slice low-calorie bread; 1 frankfurter; 1 sliced tomato; ½ cup fresh pineapple slices; no-calorie beverage.

DINNER, 420 calories:
½ cup skim or low-fat milk; 4 oz. broiled lean beef steak; baked potato without skin; 1 tablespoon sour cream; ¼ cup blueberries.

TOTAL CALORIES: 1,005

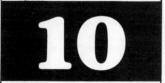

10

BREAKFAST, 255 calories:
½ cantaloupe or honeydew melon; ¼ cup cottage cheese; 2 slices bacon cooked crisp; 1 slice low-calorie bread or toast; 1 teaspoon low-calorie margarine or 1 tablespoon low-calorie jelly;

no-calorie beverage.

LUNCH, 375 calories:
Pineapple Chicken Salad[10]; 2 lettuce leaves; 1 slice whole wheat bread; ½ cup skim or low-fat milk.

DINNER, 360 calories:
4 oz. steamed scallops; 1 slice pumpernickel bread; 1 tomato, broiled slices; ½ cup frozen French cut green beans; 1 sectioned orange with ⅓ cup black raspberries; no-calorie beverage.

TOTAL CALORIES: 990

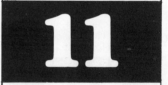

11

BREAKFAST, 210 calories:
1 apple; 1 oz. American processed cheese melted on 1 slice low-calorie bread (broiled); no-calorie beverage.

LUNCH 365 calories:
4 oz. canned salmon; 1 slice low-calorie toast; 1 pear; ½ cup winter squash, mashed; no-calorie beverage.

DINNER, 415 calories:
½ cup skim or low-fat milk; ½ green pepper, sliced; ½ cup beets; ¾ cup broiled mushrooms; 1 slice whole wheat bread; 3 oz. fried beef liver; ½ cup cherries; no-calorie beverage.

TOTAL CALORIES: 990

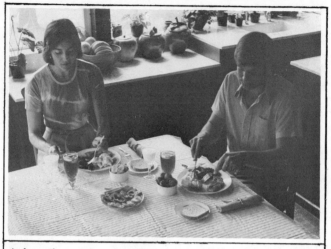

A fat-reducing diet should be centered around "calories" and "balance." There is *no food* which must be totally excluded from a sensible fat-loss diet.

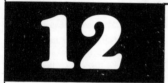

BREAKFAST, 250 calories: Scrambled Egg Special[11]; 1 slice low-calorie bread or toast; 1 teaspoon low-calorie margarine or 1 tablespoon low-calorie jelly; 4 fresh diced pineapple; no-calorie beverage.

LUNCH, 385 calories: 5 oz. lamb loin chop, broiled; 1/2 cup unsweetened apple sauce; 1 cup cauliflower (boiled or raw) with 1/4 cup American cheese, melted; 1 slice pumpernickel bread; 1/2 green pepper; 5 radishes; 1/2 cup skim or low-fat milk.

DINNER, 365 calories: 1/4 cup cottage cheese; 3/4 cup hot V-8 juice; 3 1/2 oz. broiled trout; 1 slice low-calorie bread; 1/2 cup cooked cabbage; no-calorie beverage.

TOTAL CALORIES: 1,000

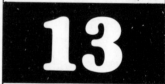

BREAKFAST, 280 calories: Potato Pancakes[12]; 1 tablespoon sour cream; 1/2 cup tomato or V-8 juice; no-calorie beverage.

LUNCH, 360 calories: Oyster Spinach Soup[13];

5 saltine crackers; 1 tomato, sliced; 2 oz. cottage cheese; no-calorie beverage.

DINNER, 360 calories:
½ cup skim or low-fat milk; Fried Chicken[14]; ½ cup asparagus; 1 tangerine, sectioned; no-calorie beverage.

TOTAL CALORIES: 1,000

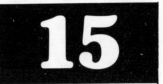

14

BREAKFAST, 255 calories:
1 orange in sections with ½ cup blueberries; 1 oz. cold cereal or ⅓ cup (uncooked) oatmeal; ½ cup skim or low-fat milk; no-calorie beverage.

LUNCH, 255 calories:
Shrimp cocktail: 12 medium/large shrimp, 3 tablespoons cocktail sauce; Broccoli-Tomato Salad[15]; ½ cup green grapes; no-calorie beverage.

DINNER, 410 calories:
¼ cup cottage cheese with 1 peach sliced; 4 oz. broiled chopped lean sirloin; 1 slice whole wheat bread; ½ tomato, sliced; no-calorie beverage.

TOTAL CALORIES: 1,005

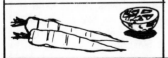

15

BREAKFAST, 275 calories:
Bacon Omelette[16]; 1 peach or plum; 1 slice low-calorie bread or toast; 1 teaspoon low-calorie margarine or 1 tablespoon low-calorie jelly; no-calorie beverage.

LUNCH, 390 calories:
Tuna Salad[17]; 1 slice low-calorie bread; 1 teaspoon low-calorie margarine; ½ cup cooked sliced beets; 1 orange, sectioned; no-calorie beverage.

DINNER, 340 calories:
½ cup skimmed or low-fat milk; 1 slice honey ham loaf; Eggplant Parmesan[18]; 1 slice low-calorie bread; ½ cup cherries; no-calorie beverage.

TOTAL CALORIES: 1,005

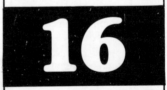

16

BREAKFAST, 265 calories:
½ cup red raspberries (fresh or unsweetened) with 1 peach, sliced; ¼ cup cottage cheese; 2 slices low-calorie bread or toast; 2 tablespoons low-calorie jelly or 2 teaspoons low-calorie margarine; no-calorie beverage.

LUNCH, 370 calories:
Grilled Swiss cheese
sandwich: 1 oz. Swiss cheese,
1 teaspoon low-calorie
margarine; 2 slices
low-calorie bread; Broccoli
Soup[19]; 2 carrot and 2 celery
sticks; no-calorie beverage.
DINNER, 370 calories:
4 oz. fish (red snapper);
1 tablespoon lemon juice;
Mashed Potatoes[20]; 1/2 cup
broiled mushrooms; 1/2 green
pepper, sliced; 5 radishes;
1 banana; no-calorie
beverage.
TOTAL CALORIES: 1,005

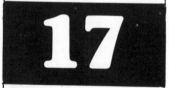

BREAKFAST, 285 calories:
1 oz. cold cereal or 1/3 cup
(uncooked) oatmeal; 3 tablespoons raisins; 1/2 cup skim or
low-fat milk; 1/2 cup fresh
diced pineapple; no-calorie
beverage.
LUNCH, 365 calories:
4 oz. fresh crabmeat; 1 tablespoon cocktail sauce; 1 cup
blueberries; 1/2 cup frozen
French cut beans (uncooked);
1 slice whole wheat bread;
2 oz. pot or farmer cheese;
no-calorie beverage.
DINNER, 350 calories:
1 cup beef bouillon with
1/4 cup mushroom slices;
1/2 cup white rice; 4 oz.

leg of lamb, lean, 1/2 cup
cooked carrots; 1 sliced
peach; no-calorie beverage.
TOTAL CALORIES: 1,000

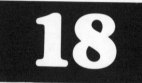

BREAKFAST, 260 calories:
Western Egg[21]; 1 slice low-
calorie bread or toast; 1 teaspoon low-calorie margarine;
1/2 grapefruit, broiled;
1/2 tomato, sliced; no-calorie
beverage.

LUNCH, 380 calories:
4 oz. broiled veal chop, fat
removed; 1/2 cup asparagus;
1 slice low-calorie bread;
1/2 cup green grapes;
no-calorie beverage.

DINNER, 360 calories:
1/2 can chunky clam chowder
soup; 1 slice rye bread; 1 oz.
pot cheese; 1 cup green
beans; 1/2 cantaloupe; 1/2 cup
skim or low-fat milk.
TOTAL CALORIES: 1,000

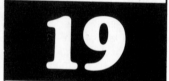

BREAKFAST, 255 calories:
Grilled Swiss cheese sandwich: 1 oz. Swiss cheese;
2 slices low-calorie bread;
1 teaspoon low-calorie

margarine; no-calorie beverage.

LUNCH, 395 calories:
Summer Salad (refer to recipe #1); 1 slice low-calorie bread; 4 oz. roasted turkey (fat removed); ½ cup skim or low-fat milk.

DINNER, 350 calories:
Raw vegetable salad: 1 carrot in strips; 2 celery sticks; 5 radishes; 2 ripe olives; ½ cup cauliflower; 4 oz. chicken livers, simmered; with ½ cup mushrooms and ½ cup onions; ½ grapefruit; no-calorie beverage.

TOTAL CALORIES: 1,000

rye bread; ½ cup broccoli with 1 tablespoon lemon juice; ½ honeydew or cantaloupe; no-calorie beverage.

TOTAL CALORIES: 1,000

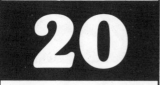

20

BREAKFAST, 265 calories:
½ grapefruit or ½ cup grapefruit juice; ¼ cup cottage cheese; 2 slices bacon cooked crisp; 1 slice low-calorie bread or toast; 1 teaspoon low-calorie margarine or 1 tablespoon low-calorie jelly; no-calorie beverage.

LUNCH 395 calories:
Shrimp Salad[22]; ½ can tomato soup, (made with water), sprinkle ½ oz. Swiss cheese in soup; 1 slice low-calorie bread, toasted; ½ cup cherries; no-calorie beverage.

DINNER, 340 calories:
4 oz. roasted turkey; 1 slice

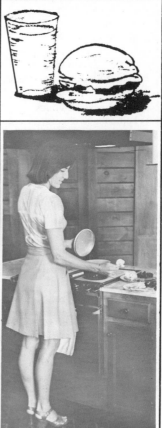

Cauliflower, raw or boiled, is an excellent low-calorie vegetable. It contains about 20 calories per serving.

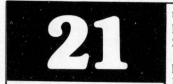

21

BREAKFAST, 275 calories:
1 peach, sliced; 1 poached egg; Hash Brown Potatoes [23]; 1 slice low-calorie bread or toast; 1 teaspoon low-calorie margarine or 1 tablespoon low-calorie jelly; no-calorie beverage.

LUNCH, 370 calories:
3/4 cup cottage cheese; 1/2 cup green beans; 1 slice low-calorie bread; 1 frankfurter; 1 tomato, sliced; 1/2 cup fresh pineapple slices; no-calorie beverage.

DINNER, 355 calories:
8 oz. broiled clams with 2 tablespoons soy sauce; 1/2 cup white rice, ready to serve; 1/2 cup skim or low-fat milk; 1/2 cup cooked collard or other type greens.

TOTAL CALORIES: 1,000

22

BREAKFAST, 235 calories:
1/2 cup flavored yogurt; 1 slice low-calorie bread or toast; 1 teaspoon low-calorie margarine or 1 tablespoon low-calorie jelly; 1 cup tomato or V-8 juice;

no-calorie beverage.

LUNCH, 400 calories:
2 bologna slices, sauteed; 1 tomato, sliced; 2 slices low-calorie bread; 1/2 cantaloupe or honeydew melon; 1/2 cup skim or low-fat milk.

DINNER, 365 calories:
3 oz. pork roast; 1/2 cup unsweetened applesauce; 1 cup yellow crook neck squash, sliced and cooked; 1/2 cup brussels sprouts; 1 tangerine, sectioned; no-calorie beverage.

TOTAL CALORIES: 1,000

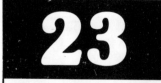

23

BREAKFAST, 260 calories:
1 orange or 1/2 cup orange juice; 2 slices French toast, (see recipe #2); 1 teaspoon low-calorie margarine or 1 tablespoon low-calorie jelly or cinnamon if desired; no-calorie beverage.

LUNCH, 270 calories:
3 oz. pork roast, lean only; Spinach Salad (refer to recipe #3); 2 tablespoons Italian salad dressing, 1 slice whole wheat bread; 1 teaspoon low-calorie margarine; 1/2 cup cherries; no-calorie beverage.

DINNER, 375 calories:
1/2 cup skim or low-fat milk; 2 oz. farmer or pot cheese;

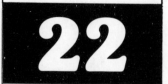

1 slice rye bread; 4 oz. flounder filet, with 1 table-spoon lemon juice; 1 baked apple; ½ cup cooked peas; no-calorie beverage.

TOTAL CALORIES: 1,005

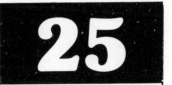

BREAKFAST, 260 calories: 1 banana; 1 oz. American processed cheese melted on 1 slice of low-calorie bread, (broiled); ½ tomato, sliced; no-calorie beverage.

LUNCH, 370 calories: Honeydew-Turkey Salad, (refer to recipe #6; 1 slice whole wheat bread; ½ cup asparagus; ½ cup skim or low-fat milk.

DINNER, 370 calories: 4 oz. broiled lean steak; 1 slice low-calorie bread toasted with 1 teaspoon low-calorie margarine; 1 cup lettuce; with 1 green pepper, diced; ½ onion, diced; 4 radishes, sliced; 2 table-spoons Italian low-calorie dressing.

TOTAL CALORIES: 1,000

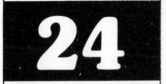

BREAKFAST, 275 calories: ½ cantaloupe or honeydew melon; 2 slices bacon, cooked crisp; 1 large egg, cooked to own preference; 1 slice low-calorie bread or toast; 1 teaspoon low-calorie margarine or 1 tablespoon low-calorie jelly; no-calorie beverage.

LUNCH, 365 calories: 4 oz. canned pink salmon, flaked over; 1 slice low-calorie toast; ½ cup winter squash, mashed; 1 banana; no-calorie beverage.

DINNER, 365 calories: ½ cup cottage cheese with 1 peach; ½ cup skim or low-fat milk; 1 slice whole wheat bread; 2 slices honey ham loaf; 1 carrot in strips; ¾ cup cooked cabbage; no-calorie beverage.

TOTAL CALORIES: 1,005

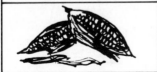

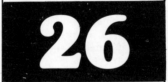

BREAKFAST, 245 calories: 1 Dominique Egg (refer to recipe #5); with 1 slice low-calorie bread and 1 teaspoon low-calorie margarine; 1 banana; no-calorie beverage.

LUNCH, 380 calories:
4 oz. roast beef on 2 slices low-calorie bread with 1 teaspoon mustard; ½ cup cooked carrots; ½ cup strawberries; no-calorie beverage.

DINNER, 370 calories:
Eggplant Parmesan (refer to recipe #18); ½ cup skim or low-fat milk; 1 slice whole wheat bread; ½ cup cooked peas; ½ cup fresh diced pineapple.

TOTAL CALORIES: 995

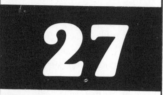

27

BREAKFAST, 280 calories:
Potato Pancakes (refer to recipe #12); top with ¼ cup unsweetened applesauce, or 1 tablespoon sour cream; ½ cup tomato juice; no-calorie beverage.

LUNCH, 375 calories:
Oyster Spinach Soup (refer to recipe #13); Swiss cheese broiled (open-face, 1 oz.) on 1 slice low-calorie bread; ½ grapefruit; no-calorie beverage.

DINNER, 345 calories:
½ cup skim or low-fat milk; 3 oz. fried liver; ½ cup fried onions; 1 slice low-calorie bread; ½ cup asparagus.

TOTAL CALORIES: 1,000

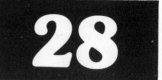

28

BREAKFAST, 235 calories:
1 oz. cold cereal or ⅓ cup (uncooked) oatmeal; ½ cup red raspberries (fresh or unsweetened); with 1 sliced peach; ½ cup skim or low-fat milk; no-calorie beverage.

LUNCH, 395 calories:
5 oz. lamb chop broiled; ½ cup unsweetened applesauce; 1 baked potato without peel; 1 slice whole wheat bread; ½ cup beets; no-calorie beverage.

DINNER, 360 calories:
1 cup sauerkraut, drained; Bar-b-que Chicken[24]; 1 slice low-calorie bread; 1 oz. farmer or pot cheese; no-calorie beverage.

TOTAL CALORIES: 1,000

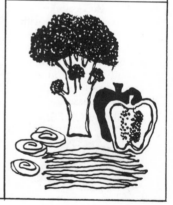

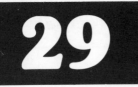

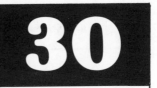

BREAKFAST, 265 calories:
½ cantaloupe or honeydew
melon; 1 oz. cheddar cheese,
grilled with 2 slices low-calorie
bread using 1 teaspoon
low-calorie margarine;
no-calorie beverage.

LUNCH, 370 calories:
2 bologna slices, sauteed;
½ cup mushrooms, sauteed
in 1 tablespoon low-calorie
margarine; 1 slice low-calorie
bread; ½ cup raspberries
mixed with 1 sectioned
tangerine; no-calorie
beverage.

DINNER, 365 calories:
4 oz. fresh crabmeat, with
1 tablespoon cocktail sauce;
½ cup frozen French cut
beans; 1 cup blueberries;
1 slice whole wheat bread;
½ cup skim or low-fat milk.

TOTAL CALORIES: 1,000

BREAKFAST, 285 calories:
Ham and Cheese Omelette[25];
1 slice low-calorie bread or
toast; 1 teaspoon margarine
or 1 tablespoon low-calorie
jelly; no-calorie beverage.

LUNCH, 375 calories:
Shrimp cocktail, 12 medium/
large shrimp with 3 tablespoons cocktail sauce;
Mushroom-Parsley Salad
(refer to recipe #8); 1 slice
pumpernickel bread; ½ cup
skim or low-fat milk; ½ cup
green grapes; no-calorie
beverage.

DINNER, 335 calories:
4 oz. lean hamburger; 1 slice
low-calorie bread; 2 leaves
lettuce; ½ tomato; ¼ cup
fresh diced pineapple;
no-calorie beverage.

TOTAL CALORIES: 995

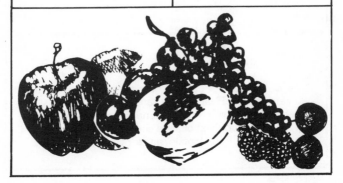

Low-Calorie Recipes

SUMMER SALAD[1]:

1 cup lettuce, shredded; 1 tomato, sliced; ¾ cup yellow crook-necked squash, sliced; ¼ cup green onion, sliced; dressing -- 1 tablespoon salad seasonings, Italian spice seasoning, and salt and pepper, plus 2 tablespoons vinegar. Mix all vegetables together. Top with dressing.

FRENCH TOAST[2]:

Dip two slices of low-calorie bread in mixture of 1 beaten egg, pinch of cinnamon, 1/8 teaspoon vanilla extract, and artificial sweetener. Using no-calorie cooking spray, brown bread on both sides. Top with low-calorie margarine, low-calorie jelly, or more cinnamon.

SPINACH SALAD[3]:

1 cup torn spinach; ½ cup sliced mushrooms; ¼ cup sliced purple onions; 2 tablespoons toasted sesame seeds. Mix vegetables together. Sprinkle sesame seeds over top.

VEAL PARMESAN[4]:

4 oz. lean veal; ½ oz. Mozzarella cheese, sliced; ⅓ cup tomato sauce. Heat tomato sauce in sauce pan using preferred seasoning. Fry veal in no-calorie cooking spray. When done, turn heat off, add cheese to veal, and cover until melted. Pour tomato sauce over top and serve.

DOMINIQUE EGG[5]:

Spread 1 slice low-calorie bread with 1 teaspoon low-calorie margarine. Cut a two-inch hole in middle of bread. In skillet, using no-calorie vegetable spray, brown both slices of bread. Then crack egg into hole of bread and cook until ready. Top egg with circle of toast.

HONEYDEW-TURKEY SALAD[6]:

½ honeydew melon, cubed; ½ cup turkey, cubed; ½ cup celery, sliced; 1 tablespoon onion, diced; 2 tablespoons low-calorie French dressing. Mix ingredients and top with French dressing.

BEEF PATTY PARMESAN[7]:

4 oz. lean hamburger; ½ oz. Mozzarella cheese, sliced; ⅓ cup tomato sauce. Heat tomato sauce in sauce pan using preferred seasoning. Fry hamburger in no-calorie cooking spray. When done, turn heat off, add cheese to burger, and cover until melted. Pour tomato sauce over top and serve.

MUSHROOM-PARSLEY SALAD[8]:

½ cup mushrooms, sliced; 1/8 cup parsley; 1/8 cup radishes, finely sliced; 1½ cups mixed greens (endive or bibb lettuce); pinch of basil, salt and pepper; 2 tablespoons low-calorie Italian dressing or wine vinegar. Combine ingredients, add seasonings, and top with dressing.

CUCUMBER-TUNA SALAD[9]:

1 small cucumber; ⅓ can or 2 oz. tuna fish; ¼ cup shredded processed American cheese; 1/8 cup chopped celery; 1 large hard-boiled egg, chopped; 1 tablespoon sweet pickle relish; 1 teaspoon onion, minced; ½ teaspoon lemon juice; paprika; salt and pepper. Cut cucumber in half length-wise and scrape out seeds. Cut a small slice from bottom of cucumber so it won't rock. Combine all ingredients and place in cucumber shells. Chill. Sprinkle with paprika and salt and pepper and serve. Makes 2 servings, 135 calories each.

PINEAPPLE-CHICKEN SALAD[10]:

½ cup chicken, cubed; 1/8 cup fresh pineapple, diced; ½ red-skinned apple, diced; ¼ cup celery, diced; 2 tablespoons raisins; salt and pepper; 1 tablespoon sour cream. Combine all ingredients, toss, and chill. Serve on salad greens.

SCRAMBLED EGG SPECIAL[11]:

1 large egg, beaten; 1 tablespoon skim or low-fat milk; 1 tablespoon green onion, sliced; 1 slice honey ham loaf (cut into bite-size pieces). Stir all ingredients together and scramble using no-calorie cooking spray.

POTATO PANCAKES[12]:

1 egg, beaten; 2 tablespoons skim or low-fat milk; 1 cup shredded potato; 2 tablespoons onion, diced; 1½ tablespoons flour; ¼ teaspoon salt; 1/8 teaspoon pepper. Combine egg and milk; add shredded potato and onion and mix. Then add flour, salt, and pepper and mix well. Using large skillet or electric griddle and no-calorie cooking spray, drop mixture by the spoonful (makes 3 to 4). Cook slowly until well browned and crisp. Turn and brown other side. Top with either sour cream or unsweetened applesauce.

OYSTER-SPINACH SOUP[13]:

1 cup skim or low-fat milk; 1 can condensed cream of chicken soup; 1, 10 oz. package frozen creamed spinach; 1, 8 oz. can of oysters, undrained; ½ cup dry white wine; pepper; lemon slices. In a large sauce pan stir milk into soup. Remove spinach from plastic pouch and add to soup. Cook and stir over medium heat, breaking up spinach until it is thawed. Simmer uncovered 10 minutes stirring occasionally. Stir in oysters, wine, and pepper. To serve, garnish with lemon slices. Makes 4 servings.

FRIED CHICKEN SPECIAL [14]:

½ chicken breast; salt and pepper; 1/8 cup bread crumbs. Season chicken breast with salt and pepper. Brown using no calorie cooking spray. Sprinkle half of bread crumbs on one side. Turn 5 minutes later and sprinkle the rest on. Cook until done.

BROCCOLI-TOMATO SALAD[15]:

1 cup fresh broccoli flowerettes; 2 tablespoons sour cream; dash of curry powder, dry mustard, seasoned salt, and pepper; 1 tomato, sliced. Cook broccoli in boiling salted water 3 to 4 minutes. Let cool. Combine sour cream and seasonings; pour over broccoli and stir to coat. Chill 2 to 3 hours. Add sliced tomato and serve on lettuce leaves.

BACON OMELET[16]:

1 egg, large; 2 slices bacon, cooked crisp and cut up; 1 tablespoon green onion, sliced; 1 tablespoon water; ½ teaspoon Worcestershire sauce; ¼ cup fresh mushrooms, sliced. Beat egg and pour into pre-heated skillet (use no-calorie cooking spray). Allow to cook until egg starts to become firm. Add rest of ingredients and cook for about a minute; turn over and continue cooking until done.

TUNA SALAD [17]:

3½ oz. tuna fish, oil drained; ¼ cup chopped celery; ¼ cup onion, chopped, 3 tablespoons cocktail sauce. Combine all ingredients and blend. Serve on lettuce leaves.

EGGPLANT PARMESAN [18]:

¾ cup eggplant, sliced; ½ cup tomato sauce; 1 oz. Mozzarella cheese, thinly sliced. Place half of eggplant on bottom of casserole dish. Cover with half of sauce and half of cheese and repeat. Cook at 400 degrees for 20 minutes.

BROCCOLI SOUP [19]:

1, 10 oz. package of frozen broccoli; 1 can condensed cream of mushroom soup; 1 can of low-fat milk; ¼ cup dry white wine; ¼ teaspoon dried tarragon; salt and pepper. In a saucepan, cook broccoli according to directions, and drain. Add soup,, milk, wine, tarragon, and salt and pepper. Heat thoroughly. Serves four.

MASHED POTATOES [20]:

1 potato, boiled and sliced; 1/8 cup skimmed or low-fat milk. Mix together and top with 1 tablespoon low-calorie margarine and salt and pepper.

WESTERN EGG [21]:

Using no-calorie cooking spray in a skillet, heat a slice of honey ham loaf on one side. Turn to other side and top with egg. Fry together to desired doneness. Place on toasted bread.

SHRIMP SALAD [22] :

1½ cups torn lettuce; 6 medium shrimp, cooked, deveined, and halved; 1 medium tomato, cut in wedges; 1 hard-boiled egg, sliced; 1 tablespoon green onion, chopped; ½ tablespoon snipped parsley; 1 tablespoon pitted ripe olives, sliced. Place lettuce in bowl. Arrange shrimp, tomatoes, egg slices, and olives over top. Serve with low-calorie dressing.

HASH BROWN POTATOES [23] :

1 cup shredded potatoes; 2 tablespoons onion, diced; salt and pepper. Mix ingredients together and put in skillet sprayed with no-calorie cooking oil. Press potatoes flat and cook until browned. Turn over and brown other side.

BAR-B-QUE CHICKEN [24] :

4 oz. roasted chicken, meat only; ¼ cup bar-b-que sauce. Place chicken in narrow pan. Cook for 20 minutes at 350 degrees. Brush sauce on top and cook until done.

HAM AND CHEESE OMELET [25] :

1 egg, large; 1 slice honey ham loaf, cut into pieces; 1 tablespoon green onion, sliced; 1 tablespoon water; ½ teaspoon Worcestershire sauce; 1 small tomato, diced; ¼ cup cottage cheese. Beat egg and pour into pre-heated skillet (use no-calorie cooking spray). Allow to cook until egg starts to become firm. Add rest of ingredients and cook for about a minute; turn over and continue cooking until done.

There are numerous ways you can plan your fat-loss diet. One desirable method is to be on a restricted intake one day (for example, 1,500, 1,200, or 1,000 calories) and eat a normal, nutritious diet on the second day. The second-day diet is equivalent to the maintenance diet you would stay on after you've lost your excess fat. Too often, after a low-calorie diet regimen, people return to their old habits and regain the excess fat.

Another approach is to make a limited reduction in the calories and stick to it longer while increasing your exercise level. Your body will gradually eliminate fatty deposits and achieve a new balance in line with your physical activity and calorie intake.

Once you've started on a diet, stick to it. "Cheating" is far more detrimental than most people think. The stimulus that tells us we're hungry comes from a center in the brain. It's turned on to make us hungry when the blood glucose level falls. Then when enough glucose is present in the cells within the appetite center, it shuts off and our hunger stops.

This center, however, can be reset. But naturally a period of training it to a new level is required. Your appetite center is adjusted to being satisfied only when the blood-glucose level peaks. You'll have recurring hunger unless the blood-glucose level is frequently increased by eating. By reducing sweets and concentrating on carbohydrates from bread, vegetable, and fruit sources, these high peak levels of glucose can be eliminated and the appetite center will be reset at a lower level.

The factors I have mentioned should be adequate for most people. If, however, you start showing any evidence of gaining fat, cut back on your calories a little. Try eliminating some of those items you don't need to provide the fundamental skeleton for a well-balanced diet. Then start increasing your level of physical activity and exercise . . . which brings us down to the next chapter . . . a very important chapter that I've titled "Proper Exercise."

Chapter 8
Proper Exercise for
Strength and Vitality

There are basically two parts to the body fat equation: calorie intake and calorie expenditure. It should be obvious that there are three ways that body fat loss or gain can be accomplished: (1) change calorie intake, (2) change calorie expenditure, or (3) change both. Too often, when attempting to lose fat, people tend to think only of reducing calorie intake (usually by some "crash diet") and to ignore the other half of the equation.

A low-calorie diet without exercise does result in weight loss. Careful studies show, however, that at least 25 percent of this weight loss (and it **can** be over 90 percent) comes not from body fat, but from the muscles, vital organs, and extracellular fluid. Loss of protein from these vital cells and organs is difficult to avoid with even small reduction in the caloric intake of an inactive person. This problem is readily overcome if a firm diet is combined with increased exercise. Additional calories are used, the physical appearance and condition is improved, and activity helps to quell the hunger pangs.

In order to get the most out of your exercise program, the exercise must be properly selected and properly performed. Just any group of exercises won't do the job.

The kind of exercise I'm talking about is not the easy toe-touching variety. Hardly! It's exercise that involves your major muscles. It's exercise that involves full-range movement. And it's exercise that makes you stronger. That's right! It makes you stronger by the workout-by-workout application of progressive resistance.

Muscles that are properly strengthened require more calories during **rest**. This is a very important fact. I repeat: **muscles that are properly strengthened require more calories at rest.**

The real problem in most cases of obesity begins with how many calories you use when you are not doing anything. The calories you use at rest under standard conditions (basal metabolism) decreases as you get older. In other words, if you eat the same number of calories you ate when you were younger and do the same amount of physical activity, you will still get fat.

Muscle cells are active cells. They are busy all the time. Fat cells are fairly inactive. They don't have nearly as many blood vessels in them as do the active muscle cells.

As we get older we tend to lose our muscle cells. There are several reasons for this, and one of these is failure to maintain physical activity of the type that strengthens the large muscles.

Therefore, a proper treatment program for obesity should not only decrease the calorie intake and increase the physical activity, but should also include measures to maintain the resting energy turnover by the body. This simply means that you need to strengthen your muscles, and keep then strong, through proper strength training. And this is true for both men and women.

Before starting a strength-training program, be sure to get the approval from your personal physician. He will probably want to give you a thorough physical examination, which includes a stress test EKG.

Proper strength training must be progressive. For our purposes, an exercise is progressive only if it involves constantly increasing workloads. The intensity of effort must be increased in proportion to increasing ability: as your muscles become stronger, they must be worked harder.

Nautilus machines provide full-range exercise for all your major muscle groups. For example, the *hip and back* machine works the buttocks and lower back, the *leg extension* strengthens frontal thighs, the *double chest* exercises the chest muscles, and the *double shoulder* works the shoulders and arms. A complete discussion of each Nautilus machine can be found in *How Your Muscles Work: Featuring Nautilus Training Equipment,* also a part of the Physical Fitness and Sports Medicine Series.

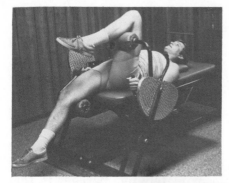

Hip and Back

Leg Extension

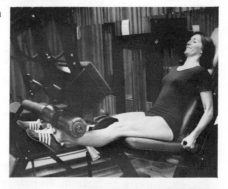

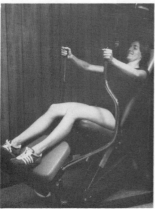

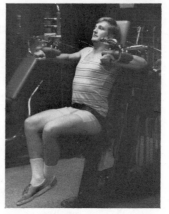

Double Chest   Double Shoulder

Progression in exercise is best accomplished by the use of barbells or weight machines, or even your own bodyweight as resistance (such as with push-ups). In other words, with each workout, you should try to add another repetition, or additional resistance.

Practical experience has shown that at least 8 repetitions should be performed, but not more than 12. When you can perform 12 repetitions in good form, that is the signal to increase the resistance by approximately five percent in that exercise at the time of the next workout.

Basic exercises should be selected that involve major muscle groups -- and where a choice exists, such exercises should involve the greatest possible range of movement. If a proper selection of exercises is made, then only a few movements are required to improve your strength and overall muscle tone.

What are the best exercises for strengthening your major muscles? Nautilus machine exercises are especially beneficial because you don't have to involve smaller, weaker muscles in working the larger and stronger torso and trunk muscles. Also, Nautilus machines provide rotary resistance, which is very important in increasing your flexibility. Some of the best Nautilus exercises are the hip and back extension, leg curl,

If Nautilus equipment is not available, conventional exercises performed with barbells should be used. Shown above from top to bottom are the *stiff-legged deadlift* for the lower back and hamstrings, the *curl* for the biceps, and the *overhead press* for the shoulders and triceps. Be sure and perform all movements in a smooth, slow manner.

Stiff-legged deadlift

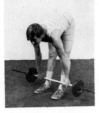

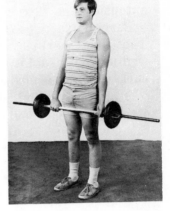

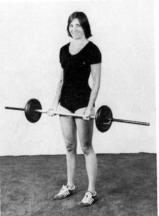

Curl

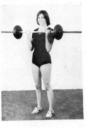

Overhead press

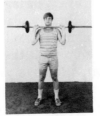

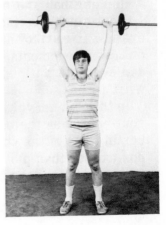

71

leg extension, pullover, shoulder shrug, neck extension and flexion, and neck rotation.

Barbell exercises can also be used effectively. The best barbell exercises are the squat, stiff-legged deadlift, standing press, standing curl, and stiff-armed or bent-armed pullover.

Other barbell and free-hand exercises that are of value are the shoulder shrug, bench press, calf raise, wrist curl . . . the chin-up on the horizontal bar (palms-up grip), the dip on the parallel bars . . . and the free-hand squat, push-up, and sit-up.

Perhaps you'd like to get started on a strength-training program, but there's no equipment available. What do you do?

First, select several large muscle exercises that require no special equipment. The free-hand squat, push-up, and sit-up are good ones. And with a little creativity you should be able to rig up a chinning bar and some type of parallel bars.

Start out by performing 8 repetitions of each exercise in good form. That may seem impossible on some movements, especially the chin-up, dip, and even the push-up. If that's the case, here's what to do.

In the chin-up, you can use your legs to help get your chin over the bar. Simply place a wooden box in front of the chinning bar and step on the box (rather than pulling up with the arms) until your chin is over the bar. Remove your feet and lower yourself very slowly (6-8 seconds). Climb back and repeat. It's a great exercise for the

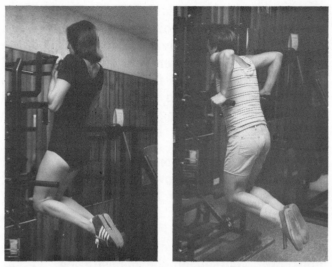

The *chin-up* on a horizontal bar and the *dip* on parallel bars are two very good exercises for the arm and torso muscles. If you're not strong enough to pull or push yourself into the top position, then use your legs (step up on a box) to assist you. Slowly lower your body to the stretched position. Climb back and repeat.

arms and back muscles. [**For building muscular strength, research has shown that the lowering portion of the exercise is far more important than the raising portion.**]

Dips on the parallel bars can be done in a similar fashion. Climb up, lock your arms (your arms should be about shoulder-width apart), and lower your body very slowly. This exercise works the chest, shoulders, and triceps. If you are unable to perform a dip in this fashion, try the push-up.

In the push-up, use your knees and lower back to help straighten your arms. Then, slowly bend your arms until your chest touches the floor and repeat.

For stomach conditioning, do sit-ups in the same (accentuate-the-lowering) fashion. With knees bent, feet securely held down, and hands on your waist, slowly lower your upper body until your back touches the floor. It's important to keep your chin tucked and shoulders rounded throughout the lowering. Once on the floor, use your arms to assist in the sitting-up movement.

The squat can be done in one of two ways. Bend your legs very slowly (you'll want to work up to 10-15 seconds lowering time in this exercise), and smoothly stand up and repeat. Or, lower your body on one leg (you may need a chair to hold on to for balance), stand up on two legs, and lower yourself on the opposite leg.

For best results from these movements, only one set of 8 to 12 repetitions, three times a week, should be done.

These five exercises (squat, chin-up, dip, sit-up, push-up), done in the accentuate-the-lowering fashion, should form your beginning strength-training program. After using these exercises for several months, you can gradually add a few barbell exercises or Nautilus machine exercises, if available.

If you are going to use barbell exercises in your program, be sure to spend the first couple of workouts practicing the movements with nothing more than an empty bar (most bars weigh 15 to 20 pounds). Stress correct form in all exercises: 2 seconds in the lifting phase and 4 seconds in the lowering phase. Fast, jerky movements are **very dangerous.** Every movement should be performed smoothly.

If you don't have access to Nautilus or conventional equipment, you should perform free-hand movements in an accentuate-the-lowering fashion. In other words, you should especially concentrate on the lowering portion of each repetition. For example, on the *squat*, *push-up*, and *sit-up*, try to take from 6 to 15 seconds to lower your body. Once you reach the bottom position, you can help yourself back to the top position. In other words, the stronger you become, the slower you should perform the downward movement.

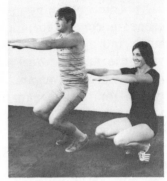

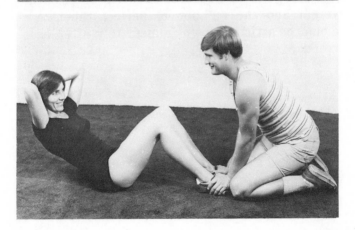

At the beginning of any strength-training program, correct form should be emphasized . . . much more than the other factors. Without proper form, your workouts become meaningless.

Therefore, in organizing a strength-training/muscle-toning program that will work hand in hand with your low-calorie diet, you should keep in mind the following guidelines:

1. Select exercises that involve large muscle groups: four to six exercises for the lower body and six to eight for the upper body.

2. Perform all repetitions in a rather slow fashion (accentuating the lowering portion of the movement) and avoid throwing or jerking actions.

3. When 12 repetitions can be performed in good form, add five percent more resistance the next exercise session and try to perform at least 8 repetitions.

4. Exercise three times a week on an every-other day schedule.

5. Keep accurate records of your progress: the weight and the number of perfect repetitions should be written down immediately after each exercise.

Chapter 9
After: Leaner and Healthier

You're probably wondering about the progress of our over-fat and out-of-shape, "before" subjects that were presented in Chapter 1? Let's take a detailed look at their results.

Sammy Johns

In working with Sammy, the first step was to introduce him to sound nutritional concepts. Instead of eating 75 percent of his food each day

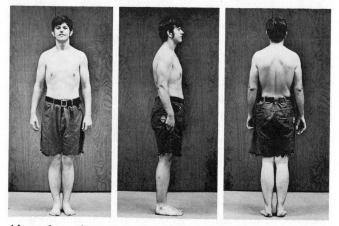

After a 6-month program of well-balanced, low-calorie meals and high-intensity exercise, Sammy Johns' body weight went from 299 pounds to 182 pounds. That's a reduction of 117 pounds of body fat.

after 5:00 p.m., Sammy was encouraged to spread his food out over four meals: breakfast, lunch, dinner, and a bed-time snack. Naturally, we reduced the quantity of food and improved the quality.

Sammy memorized the Four Basic Food Groups and I worked very closely with him on how to select food and plan meals according to the ideas presented in Chapters 6 and 7. Since Mr. Johns still lived at home with his parents, brothers, and sisters, this presented some problems . . . especially since all of them were over-fat.

I suggested that Sammy start preparing his own food. In order to accomplish this, he had to be the first up each morning so he could fix his own breakfast. After breakfast, he prepared a small lunch that usually consisted of a sandwich and a piece of fruit. He took this with him to his daily job at the Nautilus plant.

After Sammy finished work each day, instead of going home to the food and TV, he was supervised through a Nautilus exercise program three times a week and a moderate activity program on the off days. In other words, I tried to keep him busy every afternoon for about 30 minutes . . . a vigorous 30 minutes.

On Monday, Wednesday, and Friday, he performed 12 Nautilus machine exercises, progressing in each exercise in the recommended fashion. This usually took around 30 minutes to complete. On Tuesday, Thursday, and Saturday, Mr. Johns participated in one of several medium-intensity activities: fast walking, bicycling, or calisthenics. This also required about 30 minutes of his time.

Once he was home after working out, Sammy was permitted a small, well-balanced meal of not more than 400 calories. Before retiring for the night, he could have an additional 200 calories. When these meals (400 + 200 calories) were added to a 300-calorie breakfast and a 300-calorie lunch, we see that Sammy's total caloric intake each day amounted to approximately 1,200 calories.

At first, I didn't allow Sammy to drink any beer. Six weeks into the program and 30-pounds lighter, I did permit him to have an occasional beer . . . never more than one, however!

As I stated earlier, Sammy Johns was the perfect pupil. He did exactly what I told him to do, in both his eating and exercising. And he made amazing progress.

In exactly six months, Sammy lost 117 pounds of body fat. On January 1, he weighed 299 pounds . . . and on July 1, he weighed 182 pounds. That's an average fat loss of 4½ pounds per week for 26 weeks. In reality, Mr. Johns actually lost more than 117 pounds of fat since his progress in strength training revealed an almost doubling of his starting strength levels.

So, you should be able to see from Sammy Johns' facts and photos, that the optimum way to lose fat is to stimulate your body to lose fat and gain strength at the same time.

Martha Hunter

When I first met Martha Hunter, she was actively involved in the planning of a major

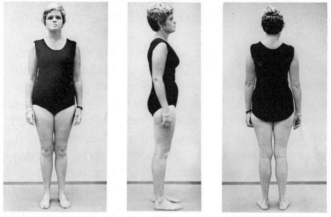

Martha Hunter's fat-reducing program consisted of a 1,000-calorie-a-day diet and supervised strength training. After three months, she had lost 22 pounds of fat and significantly increased her physical fitness.

theatrical production in Atlanta, and wanted to lose 20 pounds so she could look her best on opening night. Opening night was three months away.

Initially, Mrs. Hunter was a difficult lady to deal with. She demanded to be told exactly what to eat and drink, how often, and how much . . . as well as specifically how and how much to exercise.

To meet these needs, I worked up a 30-day, 1,000-calorie-a-day diet (see Chapter 7) for Martha to follow. I also made an effort to supervise her exercise program five days a week. To go with these factors, Martha and I established weekly exercise and dietary goals for her to strive toward. For example, we felt like she could realistically lose 1½ pounds of body fat a week. And we felt like she could make **weekly** resistance progressions in her exercises on the Nautilus machines.

Since Martha's strength-training program was only performed three times a week, we decided that during her in-between days, she should play several sets of tennis . . . or continue with the jogging program that she had previously started the year before. It was Martha's job to keep accurate records of all her exercise and eating behaviors.

The overall program progressed very well for three weeks. Having lost five pounds, she was right on schedule. Then, Martha's best friend had a party on Saturday night . . . and . . . you guessed it! Martha gained back almost all of the five pounds she'd lost.

After listening to her story on Monday morning, I looked her straight in the eyes and expressed my disappointment. Then, I promptly patted her on the back and proceeded to put her through the hardest Nautilus workout she had ever experienced.

Afterwards, I assured her that she could still accomplish her goals, and that I would help her in any way I could.

Well, this combination of factors must have worked, because Martha Hunter never faltered for the next 10 weeks.

She made her "debut" on opening night weighing 126 pounds . . . a full 22 pounds below her weight of three months earlier. During this three-month period, Martha not only lost a significant amount of body fat, but she also improved her nutritional habits, and increased her muscular strength and heart-lung efficiency. As a result, she is now playing the best tennis of her life . . . and looking quite fit.

John Kalas

Dr. John Kalas knew what his problems were, he just didn't know how to solve them. He simply did not have several hours a week to devote to exercise . . . nor did he have time to prepare his own food.

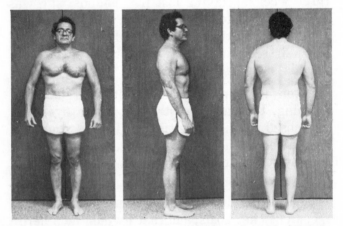

In exactly 12 months, from May 1, 1976 to April 30, 1977, Dr. John Kalas lost 51 pounds of body fat. In addition, he vastly improved his strength, flexibility, endurance, and overall health.

The big plus John did have in his favor was the fact that he didn't have any deadline to meet. He didn't have to lose 30 pounds before May 1, or be in shape for a big event July 4. We had several years, if necessary, to get him in good condition.

John and I planned his program over a 12-month period of time. We divided it into four

82

progressive steps, each step lasting three months. During the first three months, we wanted to measure the effect of **exercise only** on his blood cholesterol level, body fat percentage, and muscular strength. No changes were made in his dietary habits. John performed 10 Nautilus exercises, three times a week. The entire session lasted less than 20 minutes. During these workouts, Dr. Kalas' heart rate was closely monitored. Anytime his heart rate went over 140 beats per minute, he rested. In other words, we wanted his heart rate to stay under 140 beats per minute for the duration of the workout.

At the completion of three months of exercise only, John showed satisfactory improvements. His blood cholesterol was lower and his muscular strength was moderately improved. There was no measurable change in his percent body fat . . . especially since he was continuing to eat from 3,000 to 4,000 calories a day.

John was now ready to progress to step two. Step two of his program consisted of more intense strength training and a three-day-a-week, 1,500-calorie diet (see page 43). The three-day-a-week diet continued for six weeks; then, it was increased to seven days a week for the remaining portion of step two.

Step three introduced a three-day-a-week, 1,200-calorie diet for six weeks followed by an every day, 1,200-calorie diet for about six more weeks. The high-intensity exercise performed on Nautilus equipment was continued, except we no longer stopped an exercise when John's heart rate went over 140 beats per minute. In fact, throughout most of the workout, John's heart rate stayed between 150 and 180 beats per minute.

The last three months, step four, John adhered to a daily meal schedule of 1,000 calories. He continued with three, 20-minute Nautilus workouts a week. Two of his weekly workouts were performed in a negative-only or negative-accentuated fashion. Negative-only and negative-accentuated movements increase the intensity of the exercise. Full details of this type of training are given in my book, **Strength-Training Principles.**

By the time John Kalas' four-step program was completed, which took exactly 12 months, the following physiological changes had occured:

1. Lost 51 pounds of body fat.
2. Gained 10 pounds of muscle mass.
3. Net loss of 41 pounds of body weight.
4. Doubled muscular strength in major muscle groups.
5. Increased flexibility.
6. Lowered waking heart rate from 78 to 48 beats per minute.
7. Increased work capacity.
8. Decreased blood cholesterol level from above normal to below normal.
9. Improved posture.
10. Ability to relax markedly increased.

In writing this book on **How to Lose Body Fat** for the Physical Fitness and Sports Medicine Series, I had to limit myself to the writing of brief, concise chapters. On the one hand, this is good because we quickly get down to the "meat of the situation," with emphasis on facts not frills. On the other hand, this is bad because in dealing with generalized facts, many fine points (or exceptions) must be left uncovered. All of our authors recognize this drawback, and they hope (as I do) that the reader can effectively "read between the lines."

My original planning led me to believe that everything could be said in 9 brief chapters. When these chapters were completed, I xeroxed a dozen copies and began passing them out to my middle-aged friends. With few exceptions, their comments were similar: " . . . brief, factual . . . believable and to the point. However, I had several questions from each chapter that were left unanswered."

After carefully considering all their thoughts, I decided to include a tenth chapter. Naturally, I've called it "Questions and Answers." Hopefully, the answers to these questions will make your job of "reading between the lines" a lot easier.

Chapter 10
Questions and Answers

Why do so many people resort to fad diets?

A fad diet is any currently popular "crash" diet designed for quick weight loss and seldom supervised by a doctor. Usually the dieter eats a high proportion of one category of food. In other words, a fad diet excludes some nutrients necessary for maintaining a healthy body while losing weight.

For the last several years, dieting has become a way of life for millions of Americans. It's hardly surprising when you realize that our mass-media society glamorizes youth, vitality, and fashion-plate figures for both men and women.

Most dieters probably realize that it's dangerous to diet without medical supervision; but, the well-planned diet of the nutrition-oriented physician limits weight loss between one and two percent of the dieter's body weight per week. Is it any wonder that the woman attempting to lose 30 pounds in six weeks, so that she can appear at her daughter's wedding in a size-ten dress, strikes out on her own with the help of several magazine articles? I'm sure you're familiar with the promises on the covers of many women's magazines that guarantee "to take off 10 pounds in two weeks" with a diet dreamed up just to sell magazines.

The sad truth is that there is no quick, safe way to lose body fat. There are, indeed, ways of taking off fat more quickly than other ways, but these methods must certainly be used under close medical supervision. Drastic measures very often produce drastic results; and unless your chemistry is closely checked during drastic diets, it's quite possible for you to end up with serious damage to your vital organs.

Are there certain screening tests that I should get from my personal physician before beginning your diet and exercise program?

Yes, it's always a good idea to check with your personal physician before beginning any diet or exercise program. He may want to perform some of the following screening tests:

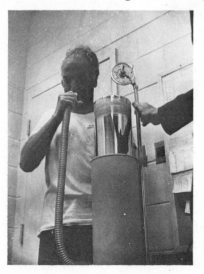

An evaluation of the mechanical properties of the lungs and chest wall can be determined by breathing into a steel container (spirometer).

(1) measurement of serum cholesterol and triglycerides, (2) hematocrit, (3) determination of serum uric-acid levels, (4) complete urine analysis, (5) thyroid function tests, such as T-3 and T-4, (6) measurement of two-hour postprandial glucose, (7) spirometry (breathing test), (8) chest X-ray, (9) resting EKG, and (10) stress test EKG, which includes blood pressure.

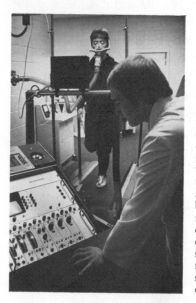

Exercise stress testing, the monitoring of one or more physiological functions during and immediately following the performance of a specific amount of exercise, is a valuable screening procedure. The test provides unique information about your heart and lung status that cannot be obtained from measurements made under resting conditions. The exercise can be performed on a stationary bicycle ergometer, a set of stairs, or as shown to the left: a motor driven treadmill.

How can I determine the calories I burn each day?

There are both direct and indirect methods. The direct methods must be done with sophisticated equipment that is not readily available to most people. One such technique measures the oxygen you breathe in and the amount of carbon dioxide you breathe out. The amount of oxygen can be converted into the number of calories your body burns. Another method actually measures the amount of heat your body produces (this is called calorimetry).

A simple method that allows you to approximate the calories you burn in a day is as follows: take your body weight in pounds, and if you are a sedentary adult, multiply it by 15. If you are an active adult, multiply your body weight by 20. Once again, these calculations will supply you with very general approximations.

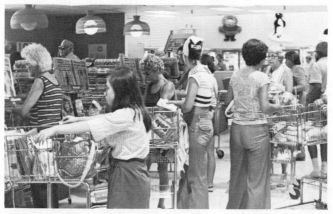

What effect does eating a high-calorie meal have on food shopping behavior? Studies have shown that obese buyers, on the average, purchase more food after a large meal. On the other hand, slim shoppers tend to buy less.

Can emotional problems contribute to my over-fat condition?

Yes, emotional problems can contribute to your over-fat condition. These problems may range from occasional nervous tension to deep-seated disturbances. You react two ways to tension: you either eat or stop eating. An interesting phenomenon is that lean people of normal weight

are usually those who, under tension, stop eating
. . . while their fatter peers tend to stuff
themselves when the going gets rough.

**When your meal schedules call for three ounces
of meat, two ounces of cheese, or some other
proportion of protein foods, I get confused. How
can I measure such small amounts?**

Purchase for yourself a small, inexpensive
scale, like a postage scale, and measure your food
on it. You'll find it quite accurate for small
amounts of food.

**Is there a way I can count calories without
actually counting calories?**

Both the energy value of the food we eat and
the energy we expend in activity are expressed in
terms of the calorie. So . . . calories do count! I

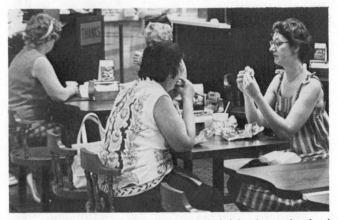

When eating in a fast-food restaurant, it's helpful to know that food
is relatively low in calories when it is thin and watery, bulky with lots
of fiber, or watery crisp instead of greasy crisp.

sympathize with you, however, concerning the use of calorie charts. They can certainly become dull nuisances.

The best I can do is offer some "ballpark" calorie values for your memorization and use. These "ballpark" figures were used in designing the dietary guidelines on page 43. These figures are purposely rounded-off to make them easier to remember: fruit juice (small) 50, egg (any style) 100, bacon slice 50, bread slice 75, potato 100, fruit 50, hard cheese (1 oz.) 100, cottage cheese (1 cup) 250, lean meat (poultry, 1 oz.) 60, regular meat (1 oz.) 80, green salad 0, salad dressing (Tbsp.) 100, sandwich 400, vegetables (1 cup) 100, skim milk (1 cup) 100, beer (can) 150, soda (can) 150.

On your day-on, day-off, 1,200 calorie diet that you used with Dr. Kalas, what did he eat on the off-days?

Dr. Kalas ate approximately 2,000 calories on his off-days. In other words, he simply added 800 calories (in snacks and second helpings) to his basic 1,200 calorie diet.

Why do I always have the greatest weight loss at the beginning, regardless of what diet I start on?

The primary reason for this quick weight loss is because you are eliminating excess fluid from your body. And for your information, a gallon of water weighs slightly more than eight pounds.

Should I take vitamin pills when I'm on your diet?

The diets recommended in this book have all been designed to provide well-balanced, low-calorie nutrition for most adult Americans. Your body has certain self-regulating mechanisms within it and will not use nutrients that are not needed, so you may be wasting considerable money by taking vitamin pills that your system doesn't need. Furthermore, only a physician should decide just which vitamins and how many units of it you need.

I lose weight for a while and then seem to hit a plateau. Why?

Anyone who has dieted frequently has experienced the "weight plateau." In most cases, this is a temporary phenomenon, and after a few weeks you will once again begin to lose weight on a low-calorie diet. Evidently, certain people tend to occasionally retain fluid as they lose fat. Thus, even though they are losing fat, it doesn't show on the scales . . . at least not for several weeks.

Then, there are some people with unusual muscular potential who can actually stimulate muscular growth at the same rate as they are losing body fat. In other words, over a two-week period of time, such a person might lose five pounds of fat and gain five pounds of muscle. While his bodyweight would remain the same, his overall appearance would be changing for the better.

I feel bloated and always gain weight just before my period. What can I do about this?

Fluid retention in obesity is not an unusual occurence. Fluid retention in women prior to the beginning of a menstrual period is also common. When this fluid retention occurs, bodyweight shifts in a given month may range from two to three pounds to as much as six to ten pounds. Simply limiting the amount of salt in your diet can often eliminate this problem. In some cases, however, the reasons for excessive fluid retention are more complex. Only your physician can tell for sure.

Is it okay to skip a meal occasionally?

No! Many people who do skip meals have the tendency to nibble later on or overeat at the next meal and actually end up consuming more calories for the day.

How much water should I drink on your diet?

If you are healthy, you can drink as much water as you wish. You will not have a fluid retention problem from drinking water, if at the same time you don't take in excessive amounts of salt. Remember, the more water you drink, the more you will eliminate, providing you have normal kidneys and a normal heart.

I need all the help I can get when I'm on a reducing diet. Can you suggest any "crutches?"

Here's a few things you can do to obtain oral

gratification at low-calorie costs:

1. Chew sugarless gum
2. Drink ice water
3. Drink a diet soda
4. Munch on carrot or celery sticks
5. Go for a walk
6. Do some vigorous exercise
7. Call a friend on the phone.

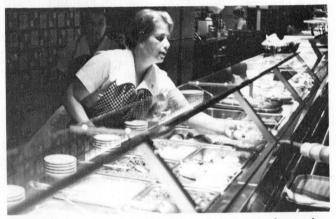

Eating out doesn't have to be a "no no" on your reducing diet. Cafeterias, many times, can be a good source of well-balanced, low-calorie food. Remember, to choose one small serving from each of the four food groups.

Recently I read where a leading nutritionist recommended a reducing diet composed of six small meals a day. Is this a good idea?

The important issue is not how many times a day you eat, but your nutritional record once your foods have been totaled for the day. In other words, has your 24-hour food consumption been adequate? Is the distribution of your calories throughout the day such that you burn up as many calories as you take in?

There's nothing wrong with more than three meals a day, even as many as six. Many dieters, in fact, prefer to spread out their caloric allowance this way. As long as your total caloric intake is what you need -- and no more -- it's fine.

How often should I weigh myself when I'm on your training program?
Even though you may register a few unexplained gains (some people tend to retain water for a while during fat loss; pre-menopausal women retain some water every month before menstruation), there is merit in weighing yourself every day and plotting the weight on a chart. You should find it encouraging to note a slow, steady decline in your body weight.

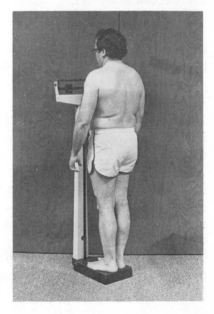

Make sure your body weight is accurately measured at the same approximate time each day.

What about the use of diuretics in a fat-loss program?

I can not recommend diuretics as a part of a fat-loss program. Diuretics are chemical substances to rid the body of excessive water. You must remember, however, that there is very little water in fat. Thus, the weight you lose from diuretics is not from fatty deposits.

People who self-administer diuretics can become depleted of potassium and other substances. If too much potassium is lost, blood pressure may drop, and serious problems can occur. In addition, overuse of diuretics can irritate the kidneys, or even cause diabetes.

What type of diet should I use once I've lost my excess body fat?

After losing your excess body fat, you should be thoroughly familiar with the Basic Four Food Groups: meat, milk, fruit and vegetable, and bread and cereal (see pages 39-44). Each time you sit down for a meal, you should try to select **one small** serving of food from each of these groups. Additional foods from the "other food" group can help add more calories to your meals.

Generally speaking, a good maintenance diet for most women should contain about 1,800 calories (slightly more for men). You can easily plan 1,800-calorie menus by simply adding seconds or snacks to the basic 1,200-calorie diet (see page 43), or you can plan higher-calorie main dishes and desserts that are ordinarily forbidden.

For my exercise program, I don't have access to Nautilus equipment. What should I do?

Alternatives to using Nautilus equipment are discussed on pages 71 and 72. Most people have access to barbells. If not, use the free-hand exercises suggested on pages 73 and 74.

There are many other forms of exercise that can be employed . . . like bicycling, swimming, jogging, jumping rope, and tennis. While these activities do work your heart and lungs and do burn calories, they do little in the way of developing full-range strength in your major muscles.

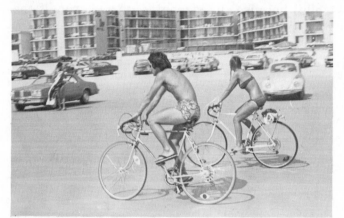

Bicycling offers an excellent way to condition the heart and lungs. For best results in losing body fat, however, bicycling should be combined with strength training.

Try your best to make a progressive, three-day-a-week, strength-training program the "meat and potatoes" of your weekly exercise.

I'm a 30-year old female and stand 5'5" and weigh 139 pounds. I figure I have about 12 to 15

pounds of body fat to lose. But won't the heavy exercise you recommend make my muscles larger and more masculine looking?

No! Most women could not develop large muscles if their lives depended on it.

A small percentage of women, less than one percent, do have large muscles . . . particularly in their legs. This is either inherited, or results from an above-average amount of the male hormone in the system. The adrenal glands and the sex glands, of both men and women, secrete small amounts of the non-dominant hormone.

Heavy exercise (strength training) is worthwhile because it strengthens and conditions your muscles, which enhances athletic ability, burns more calories at rest, and facilitates other

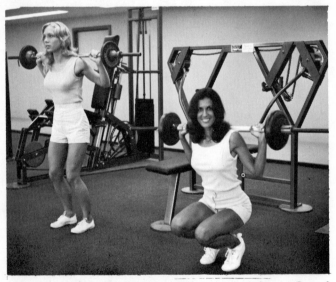

Stronger muscles will definitely improve a woman's figure. One of the best conventional exercises for the hips and legs, the barbell squat, is pictured above.

activities, from house work to having a baby. And the stronger your muscles become, the more physically attractive you'll be.

Even though I'm fairly slim, I've got large fatty deposits on the sides of my upper thighs. Are there exercises I can do to reduce them?

Spot reducing is not possible. Many women, however, believe that concentrated exercise for a body part that is laden with fat will be effective in removing the fat (spot reduction). Although exercise does play a role in the reduction of body fat (along with proper diet), it is mobilized out of the multiple fat cells all over the body.

Other factors also determine the way in which fat is distributed over your body. The most important of these is **inherited**. Just as different races and different families have characteristic height, coloring, and nose shapes, they may have characteristic patterns of fat distribution. Thus, it appears that you've inherited the potential (probably from your mother) to store fat on your upper thighs. Try as you may, you can't change it. Even if you lose a significant amount of body fat, you'll still be disproportionately fat in your upper thighs. This does not mean that proper exercise won't benefit you. Proper exercise will strengthen your hip and leg muscles, and the fat and skin that surround these muscles will become tighter and firmer.

When I reduce I always lose fat from my breasts. Can anything be done to prevent this?

If you lose fat at a rate not exceeding five

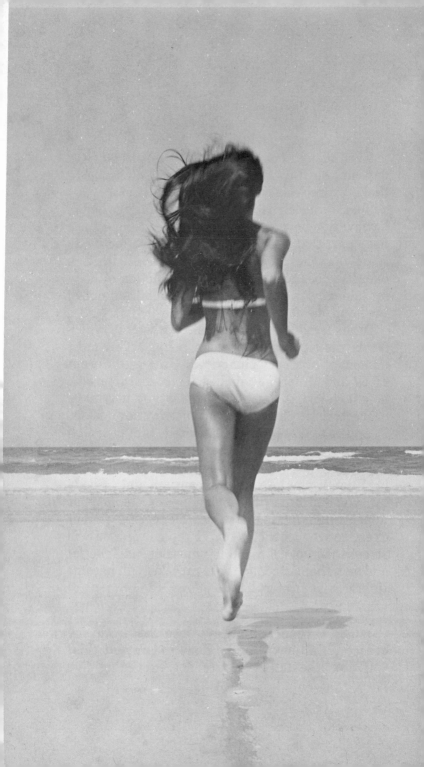

pounds per month, and if you simultaneously do exercises that firm your breasts, you should not lose a disproportionate amount of fat from that area. In fact, you should actually be able to improve the shape and firmness of your breasts with proper exercise.

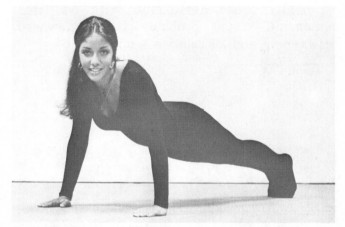

A good free-hand exercise for firming and shaping your bustline is the push-up performed in an accentuate-the-lowering fashion. For best results, take from 6 to 12 seconds to lower yourself.

How can I find out how many calories I burn during exercise?

The answer to this question depends on your age, sex, body weight, and several other factors. Dr. Frank Konishi has published a book (see bibliography) that fully discusses these factors. He presents tables and charts on various

The woman on the left has been involved in a heavy resistance, strength-training program for over 18 months. She regularly trains with over 100 pounds on the Nautilus leg machines, and at a body weight of 119 pounds she can perform 9 continuous chin-ups. Remember, stronger muscles will help you lose fat because they enable you to burn more calories at rest.

activities that I'm sure you'll find helpful. As a rough estimate, however, we find that walking briskly requires 5.2 calories per minute, bicycling consumes 8.2 calories per minute, jogging takes 10 calories a minute, and swimming uses up 11.2 calories a minute. Strength-training exercises, especially those performed with Nautilus equipment, would probably fall somewhere between 15 and 20 calories a minute.

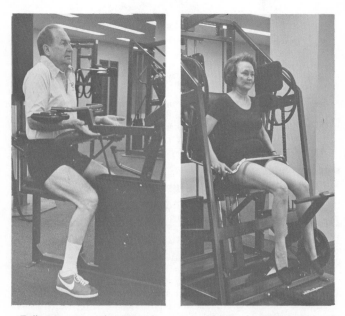

Full-range strength training burns more calories per minute than any other activity. And practiced properly, it can benefit almost any age group from 8 to 80. Shown above is a shoulder shrug and pullover being performed on Nautilus machines.

Is there any special exercise that will eliminate my double chin? I'm full-faced and I've always had this problem. Recently, however, it seems to be getting worse.

Evidently you have an extra large fat pad under your chin. In other words, you have more fat cells under your chin than the average person. From a previous question and answer, I pointed out that spot reducing is a myth. Even after having reduced your overall percentage of body fat, you will still have a considerable amount of fat under your chin. Remember, how you store fat is basically a family characteristic.

There are no special exercises that will eliminate the fat from under your chin or that will change how you store fat. In addition, the mechanical vibrating straps you frequently see in health spas are totally unproductive.

Your best bet is to reduce your overall body fat (get as lean as possible) and strengthen the major muscles of your shoulders and neck. Thus, even though the fat will not be removed, it will hang differently.

What about the wide variety of spot-reducing gadgets that are highly advertised? Are you saying that none of them work?

That's exactly what I'm saying. Not only do they not result in permanent fat loss, but many of the gadgets are dangerous. Let's examine some of the most popular ones:

1. Motorized exercycles. -- An exercycle is a motorized bicycle that moves your legs and torso

for you. Since the machine is pulling your legs up and down, it is doing the work, not you.

2. Electrical shock. -- This machine supposedly makes muscles contract involuntarily through small electric charges. Actually the muscle movements are too small to consume enough energy to cause a noticeable reduction in fat. And doctors believe certain of these machines can be dangerous to the heart and other organs that can respond to electrical stimuli.

3. Vibrating belts. -- A mechanical vibrating belt may relax you and make you feel better, but it certainly won't remove the fat. Fat cannot be shaken, tickled, beaten, or stroked from your body.

4. Rubber clothes. -- These clothes, which range from belts, shorts, and shirts to full outfits, are supposed to make you "sweat off" the fat and inches. Any weight you lose is simply a result of dehydration, which is quickly replaced when you quench your thirst. And none of the water you lose when you sweat comes from your body fat, since fat contains just a small percentage of water.

5. Sauna wraps. -- In this principle, your body (or the specific part you want reduced) is wrapped with tape, which has been soaked in a "secret" solution. You then sit in a sauna bath for 30 minutes, and supposedly the secret solution draws the excess fat from your body. Again, you can't passively sweat fat off your body.

6. "Cellulite" remedies. -- Cellulite is supposedly a unique type of fat that can only be removed by a costly and elaborate program. This

is simply not true. Fat is fat whether it's dimpled, bumpy, or looks like orange peel. In fact, the American Medical Association has issued a statement calling cellulite a hoax and denouncing its remedies as economic exploitation.

Will losing fat make me more physically fit?
It's very important to point out that a person who loses fat does not automatically become more physically fit. An over-fat, sloppy, and unfit person who loses 25 pounds of fat from diet only, is simply less fat and still sloppy and unfit.

Well-balanced, low-calorie diets should always be combined with progressive exercise. Losing fat should go hand-in-hand with building strength and muscle toning.

•••••

In conclusion, I would like to re-emphasize that losing body fat is hard . . . very hard! In this book, I've offered no magic formulas, no easy solutions, no painless pills. Instead, I've provided you with a sound, sensible approach: a well-balanced, low-calorie diet combined with high-intensity exercise. This approach does work . . . fat is removed slowly, muscles are toned and strengthened, and your health is improved. But it takes discipline and patience, as well as the proper know-how.

This book has given you the **know-how**. You must supply the **discipline** and **patience**.

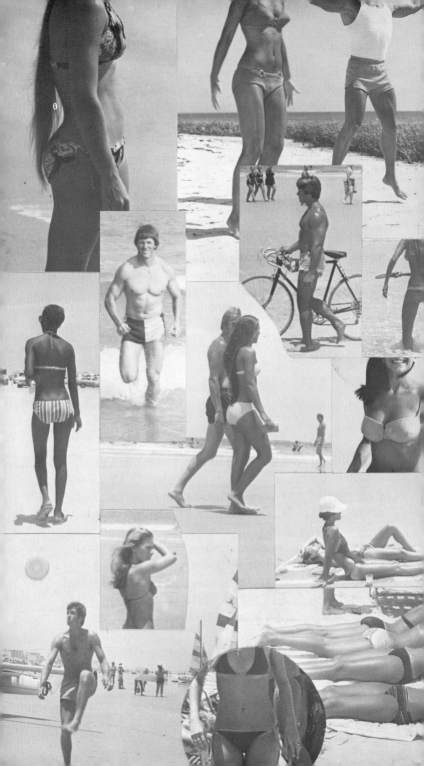

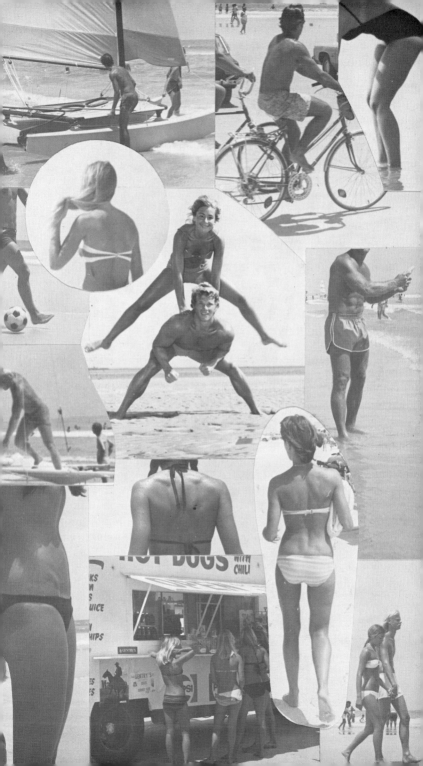

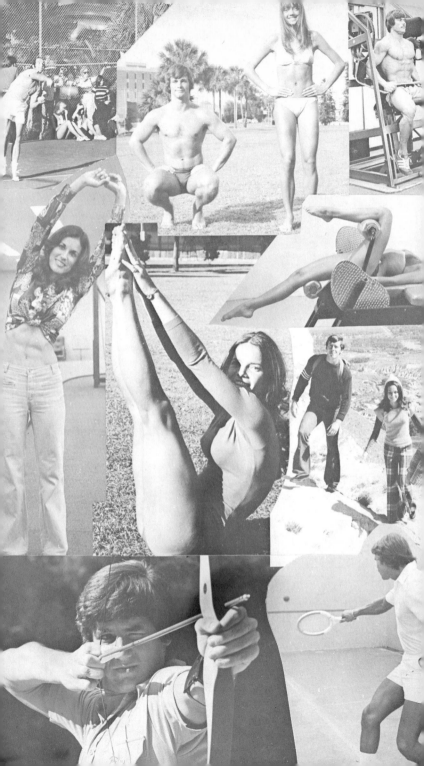

Bibliography

Antonetti, Vincent. **The Computer Diet**. New York: M. Evans and Co., 1973.

Berland, Theodore. **Consumer Guide's Rating the Diets**. Stokie, Illinois: Publications International, Ltd., 1974

Consumer Affairs Committee, Americans for Democratic Action. "Drug Companies Get Fat on People's Desire to Lose Weight," (Printed report). January 19, 1976.

Consumer Guide's The Brand Name Food Game. Stokie, Illinois: Publications International, Ltd., 1974.

Council on Food and Nutrition of the American Medical Association. "A Critique of Low-Carbohydrate Ketogenic Weight Reduction Regimens -- A Review of Dr. Atkins' Diet Revolution." **Journal of the American Medical Association** 224: 1415-19, June 4, 1973.

Darden, Ellington. **Strength-Training Principles**. Winter Park, Florida: Anna Publishing, Inc., 1977.

Darden, Ellington. **Olympic Athletes Ask Questions About Exercise and Nutrition**. Winter Park, Florida: Anna Publishing, Inc., 1977.

Darden, Ellington. **Nutrition and Athletic Performance**. Pasadena, California: The Athletic Press, 1976.

Deutsch, Ronald M. **The Family Guide to Better Food and Better Health**. New York: Bantam Books, 1973.

Hirschi, Jules, and Knittle, Jerome L. "Cellularity of Obese and Non-obese Human Adipose Tissue." **Federation Proceedings 29:** 1516-1521, 1970.

How to Feed Your Family to Keep Them Fit and Happy . . . No Matter What. New York: Golden Press, 1972

Konishi, Frank, and Harrison, Sharon L. "Body Weight-Gain Equivalents of Selected Foods." **Journal of the American Dietetic Association** 70: 365-68, April 1977.

Konishi, Frank. **Exercise Equivalents of Foods**. Carbondale: Southern Illinois University Press, 1974.

Labuza, Theodore P. **The Nutrition Crisis: A Reader**. St. Paul: West Publishing Co., 1975.

Lamb, Lawrence E. **Metabolics**. New York: Harper and Row. 1974.

Mann, George V. "Obesity, the National Spook." **American Journal of Public Health** 61: 1491-98, August 1971.

Mayer, Jean. **A Diet For Living**. New York: Pocket Books, 1977.

Mayer, Jean. **Overweight**. Englewood Cliffs, New Jersey: Prentice-Hall, 1968.

110

Nelson, Ralph A. **et. al.** "Psychology and Natural History of Obesity." **Journal of the American Medical Association** 223: 627-630, 1973.

Shephard, Roy J. **Alive Man!** Springfield, Illinois: Charles C. Thomas, 1972.

Solomon, Neil. **The Truth About Weight Control**. New York: Dell Publishing Co., 1971.

Stare, Frederick, and Witschi, Jelia C. "Diet Books: Facts, Fads and Frauds." **Medical Opinion** 1: 13-18, 1972.

Texas Dietetic Association Diet Manual. Houston: Texas Dietetic Association, 1976.

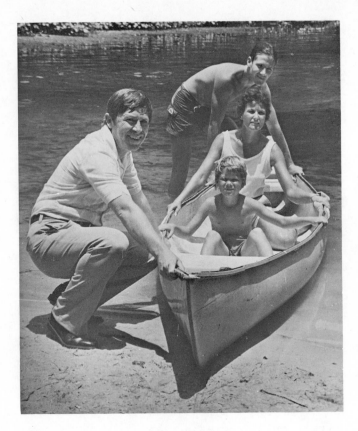

"Dr. Darden's book exposes many of the 'Lose Now — Regain Later' crash diets while providing a medically-sound plan for removing excess body fat. My family and I feel that this program can make a valuable contribution to your health and well-being."

William E. Pate, M.D.
Chief of Staff,
West Volusia Memorial Hospital
DeLand, Florida